Alternate Therapies in the Treatment of Brain Injury and Neurobehavioral Disorders
A Practical Guide

T0256258

Alternate Therapies in the Treatment of Brain Injury and Neurobehavioral Disorders
A Practical Guide

Gregory J. Murrey, PhD, LP, ABPN
Editor

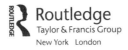

Routledge
Taylor & Francis Group
New York   London

First published by The Haworth Press, Inc.

This edition published 2013 by Routledge

Routledge	Routledge
Taylor & Francis Group	Taylor & Francis Group
711 Third Avenue	2 Park Square, Milton Park
New York, NY 10017	Abingdon, Oxon OX14 4RN

Routledge is an imprint of the Taylor & Francis Group, an informa business

Identities and circumstances of individuals discussed in this book have been changed to protect confidentiality.

Cover design by Lora Wiggins.

Library of Congress Cataloging-in-Publication Data

Alternate therapies in the treatment of brain injury and neurobehavioral disorders : a practical guide / Gregory J. Murrey, editor.
    p. cm.
    Includes bibliographical references and index.
    ISBN-13: 978-0-7890-2134-2 (hard : alk. paper)
    ISBN-10: 0-7890-2134-X (hard : alk. paper)
    ISBN-13: 978-0-7890-2135-9 (soft : alk. paper)
    ISBN-10: 0-7890-2135-8 (soft : alk. paper)
    1. Brain damage—Alternative treatment. 2. Brain damage—Patients—Rehabilitation. 3. Neurobehavioral disorders—Alternative treatment. 4. Neurobehavioral disorders—Patients—Rehabilitation.
    [DNLM: 1. Brain Injuries—rehabilitation. 2. Cognition Disorders—rehabilitation. 3. Complementary Therapies—methods. WL 354 A466 2005] I. Murrey, Gregory J. (Gregory Jay), 1960-

RC387.5.A498 2005
616.8'046—dc22

                                        2005004565

CONTENTS

ABOUT THE EDITOR

Gregory J. Murrey, PhD, LP, ABPN, is on the clinical faculty of the Fielding Graduate Institute and has directed the rehabilitation program of the Minnesota Neurorehabilitation Hospital, which serves patients with traumatic brain injury (TBI) and associated behavioral disorders. He not only holds a PhD in clinical psychology but has also completed specialized training in clinical neuropsychology at Duke University Medical Center. He has extensive experience in the evaluation and treatment of persons with TBI. Dr. Murrey has presented and published widely on the subject of TBI rehabilitation.

CONTRIBUTORS

Margaret E. Ayers, MA, is the owner and president of Neuro-pathways EEG Imaging, Inc., in Beverly Hills, California. She is board certified by the Biofeedback Society of America. She has extensive training and experience in the clinical applications of EEG feedback in various patient populations, and has published extensively in the area.

Wendy Magee, PhD, is the head of music therapy at the Royal Hospital for Neuro-Disability in London, England. She has extensive experience in the clinical application of music therapy modalities with various medical and neurological patient populations.

Martha A. Murrey, MA, CCC-SLP, received her master's degree in speech language pathology from Washington State University. She is currently in private practice in Brainerd, Minnesota, and specializes in treatment of persons with stroke, traumatic brain injury, and swallowing disorders.

Duane A. Reynolds, BA, LSW, LADC, BCCR, is the associate executive director of the Vinland Center in Minnesota, which provides specialized chemical-dependency treatment to persons with traumatic brain injury.

Susan Schaefer, MS, CCC-SLP, has served as a speech pathologist consultant to the laryngectomee association with the American Cancer Society and as director of rehabilitation, developing a coma-management program to promote recovery of long-term brain-injured patients. More recently, she has developed a rural-based multi-regional rehabilitation program in southwest Missouri. She specializes in the areas of swallowing, cognitive/linguistic rehabilitation, and language.

Mark Sell, RT, is the coordinator of the community integration, therapeutic recreation, and art therapy programs at the Minnesota Neurorehabilitation Hospital.

Ann Wedel, PTR, HTR, is a physical therapist and co-coordinator of the horticultural therapy program at the Minnesota Neurorehabilitation Hospital, which serves patients with traumatic brain injury and associated neurobehavioral disorders. She is trained in a variety of alternative therapeutic interventions including craniosacral therapy, biofeedback, herbal therapies, and aromatherapies.

Barbara Wheeler, MT-BC, is on the music therapy faculty at the University of Kentucky–Louisville. She is board certified in music therapy.

Acknowledgment

A special thanks to Arlene Jones, who patiently and diligently provided transcription support in the development of this text.

Chapter 1

Introduction and Overview of Brain Injury in Executive Dysfunction

Gregory J. Murrey

Most therapy professionals have become increasingly aware of the prevalence of traumatic brain injuries (TBIs) in the general population and their corresponding adverse effects on the functioning and mental health of individuals with such injuries. Although the actual prevalence of TBI in the general population is not known (Burg et al., 1996), the estimated prevalence in the U.S. general population is 390 per 100,000 or 0.39 percent (Guerrero et al., 2000). Although the clinical and functional effects vary widely and are unique with each individual, the professional literature offers much information on the clinical sequelae associated with TBI (Ben-Yishay and Silver, 1997; Hammond et al., 2001; Mooney and Speed, 2001; Sander et al., 2001; Steadman-Pare et al., 2001; Williams et al., 2002).

Persons who have suffered TBI to the frontal temporal regions of the brain often present with significant deficits in executive functioning with resulting neurobehavioral disorders (Grace et al., 1999; Sohlberg et al., 1993, Trudel et al., 1998; Prigatano, 1999). These neurobehavioral disorders typically include disturbances in initiation, impulse control, attention and memory functions, sequencing, problem solving, planning, self-monitoring, and frustration tolerance (Goldstein and Levin, 1995; Lezak, 1993; Prigatano, 1999). As a result of these deficits, many persons with brain injury present with physical and verbal aggression and other inappropriate social behaviors (Sohlberg et al., 1993; Hart and Jacobs, 1993; Varney and Menefee, 1993) that lead to failures in community residential and vocational settings (Wehman et al., 1995; Buffington and Malec, 1997; Jacobs, 1997; Sander et al., 1997). In addition, many of these persons have significant deficits in planning and initiating leisure activity (Lezak, 1993). More recent studies by the Minnesota State Department of Health confirm not only the high incidence of TBI within the state (Minnesota Department of Health, 2001) but also the significant number of persons with histories of TBI being admitted to state psychiatric hospitals (Murrey et al., 2004). As a result of this increased awareness of the need for specific services for persons with TBI and associated neurobehavioral disorders, a variety of treatment models and programs have been developed among various states in an attempt to meet these needs (Digre et al., 1994; Murrey et al., 1998).

Unfortunately, prognosis and treatment success rates for persons with chronic neurobehavioral dysfunctions following TBI are not very promising. Indeed, many such persons tend to lose, burn out, or become lacking in community support and resources within just a few years after the injury. Many persons without such resources typically end up in inpatient state psychiatric facilities, homeless, or incarcerated due to legal issues related to their behavioral dysfunction. Traditional therapies (physical, occupational, and speech) are appropriate for patients with acute injuries for up to about one year following the TBI, but are typically not available (due to funding issues), not appropriate, and/or not beneficial to this chronically neurobehaviorally disordered population. Furthermore, a typical disorder that this patient population presents with is a syndrome known as *anosognosia,* or lack of awareness of deficits. This syndrome has been studied at length by neuropsychologists and neuroscientists (Prigatano, 1999; Prigatano and Schacter, 1991; Sohlberg et al., 1993; Trudel, 1998). This form of agnosia is a neurologically based syndrome that is secondary to a neurological insult, and is not a psychiatric syndrome, such as denial. Anosognosia runs along a continuum from very mild to very severe and chronic. Although anosognosia and other forms of agnosia are common following acute brain injury, depending on the severity and site or location of the brain injury it may subside or improve, or it could remain as a chronic condition. Anosognosia is typically a result of either damage to the frontal cortex/ frontal lobes of the brain or of bilateral damage to the right and left brain hemispheres. Other executive or frontal lobe dysfunctions include deficits in planning, problem solving, and impulse control as well as an inability to initiate behaviors even when the desire to do so is present. Such neurocognitive and neurobehavioral changes are often labeled as personality changes by both laypersons and professionals (Prigatano, 1999).

Thus, the successful treatment of a person with traumatic brain injury and associated severe and chronic neurobehavioral dysfunction is quite complex and can be very discouraging to the treatment team, to family members, and to the TBI patient. Standard functional measures and treatment may not be beneficial in treating this particular patient population (Murrey and Starzinski, 2004; Hammond et al., 2001; Steadman-Pare et al., 2001). Thus, clinicians have attempted to find and implement nontraditional or more atypical approaches in the treatment of this TBI patient population as a means for greater treatment success and long-term positive outcomes (Murrey et al., 2001; Murrey and Starzinski, 2004).

In the following chapters of this text, various nontraditional or atypical treatment programs, therapies, and techniques are discussed at length. Each approach promotes a holistic treatment model for this particular population. Readers will find models of therapy implementation for use within a hospital-based rehabilitation program. In addition, case examples are presented along with additional resources and/or readings related to each treatment or approach.

Many of the therapies presented are not discipline specific; clinicians from a variety of therapy and discipline backgrounds can use a given treatment or approach. However, specific and specialized training is essential. Some of the therapies require or recommend a certain level of training or certification, and others require only general expertise or experience in the given area. It should also be emphasized that many of the ultimate goals of the different therapies are the same or similar for the neurobehaviorally disordered TBI patient.

REFERENCES

Ben-Yishay, Y. and Silver, S. (1997). Relationship Between Employability and Vocational Outcomes After Intensive Holistic Cognitive Rehabilitation. *The Journal of Head Trauma Rehabilitation, 2*(10):35-38.

Buffington, A.L. and Malec, J.F. (1997). The Vocational Rehabilitation Continuum: Maximizing Outcomes Through Bridging the Gap from Hospital to Community-Based Services. *Journal of Head Trauma Rehabilitation, 12*(5):1-13.

Burg, J., McGuire, L., Burright, R., and Donovick, P. (1996). Prevalence of Traumatic Brain Injury in an Inpatient Psychiatric Population. *Journal of Clinical Psychology in Medical Settings, 3*(3):251-253.

Digre, P.D., Kamen, D., Vaughn, S., Weinand, A., and Helgeson, S. (1994). Selected States Public Policy Response to Traumatic Brain Injury. *Journal of Head Trauma Rehabilitation, 9*(2):12-26.

Goldstein, R.C. and Levin, H.S. (1995). Neurobehavioral Outcome of Traumatic Brain Injury: Coma, the Vegetative State, and the Minimally Responsive State. *Journal of Head Trauma Rehabilitation, 10*(1):57-73.

Grace, J., Stout, J.C., and Malloy, P.F. (1999). Assessing Frontal Lobe Behavioral Syndromes with the Frontal Lobe Personality Scale. *Psychological Assessment Resources, 6*(3):269-284.

Guerrero, J., Thurman, D.J., and Sniezek, J.E. (2000). Emergency Department Visits Associated with Traumatic Brain Injury: United States 1995-1996. *Brain Injury, 16*(2):181-186.

Hammond, F.D., Grattan, K.D., Sasser, H., Corrigan, J.D., Busbnik, T., and Zafonte, R.D. (2001). Long-Term Recovery Course After Traumatic Brain Injury: A Comparison of the Functional Independence Measure and Disability Rating Scale. *Journal of Head Trauma Rehabilitation, 16*(4):318-329.

Hart, T. and Jacobs, H.E. (1993). Rehabilitation and Management of Behavioral Disturbances Following Frontal Lobe Injury. *Journal of Head Trauma Rehabilitation, 8*(1):1-12.

Jacobs, H.E. (1997). The Clubhouse: Addressing Work-Related Behavioral Challenges through a Supportive Social Community. *Journal of Head Trauma Rehabilitation, 12*(5):14-27.

Lezak, M.D. (1993). Newer Contributions to the Neuropsychological Assessment of Executive Functions. *Journal of Head Trauma Rehabilitation, 8*(1):24-31.

Minnesota Department of Health (2001). Minnesota Injury Prevention Resource Guide. Minneapolis, MN: Minnesota Department of Health.

Mooney, G. and Speed, J. (2001). The Association Between Mild Traumatic Brain Injury and Psychiatric Conditions. *Brain Injury, 15*(10):865-877.

Murrey, G.J., Helgeson, S.R., Courtney, C.T., and Starzinski, D.T. (1998). State-Coordinated Services for Traumatic Brain Injury Survivors: Toward a Model Delivery System. *Journal of Head Trauma Rehabilitation, 13*(6):72-81.

Murrey, G.J. and Starzinski, D. (2004). An Inpatient Neurobehavioral Rehabilitation Program for Persons with Traumatic Brain Injury: Overview and Outcome Data for the Minnesota Neurorehabilitation Hospital. *Brain Injury, 18*(6):519-531.

Murrey, G.J., Starzinski, D.T., and LeBlanc, A.J. (2004). Base Rates of Traumatic Brain Injury History in Adults Admitted to State Psychiatric Hospitals: A 3-Year Study. *Rehabilitation Psychology, 49*(3):259-261.

Murrey, G.J., Wedel, A., and Dirks, J. (2001). A Horticultural Therapy Program for Brain Injury Patients with Neurobehavioral Disorders. *Journal of Therapeutic Horticulture, 12:*4-8.

Prigatano, G. (1999). *Principles of Neuropsychological Rehabilitation.* New York: Oxford University Press.

Prigatano, G. and Schacter, D. (1991). *Awareness of Deficit After Brain Injury: Clinical and Theoretical Issues.* New York: Oxford University Press.

Sander, A.M., Kreutzer, J.S., and Fernandez, C.C. (1997). Neurobehavioral Functioning, Substance Abuse, and Employment After Brain Injury: Implications for Vocational Rehabilitation. *Journal of Head Trauma Rehabilitation, 12*(5):28-41.

Sander, A.M., Roebuck, T.M., Struchen, M.A., Sherer, M., and High, W. (2001). Long-Term Maintenance of Gains Obtained in Postacute Rehabilitation by Persons with Traumatic Brain Injury. *Journal of Head Trauma Rehabilitation, 13*(6):356-373.

Sohlberg, M.M., Mateer, C.A., and Stuss, D.T. (1993). Contemporary Approaches to the Management of Executive Control Dysfunction. *Journal of Head Trauma Rehabilitation, 8*(1):45-58.

Steadman-Pare, D., Colantonio, A., Ratcliff, G., Chase, S., and Vernich, L. (2001). Factors Associated with Perceived Quality of Life Many Years After Traumatic Brain Injury. *The Journal of Head Trauma Rehabilitation, 16*(3):330-342.

Trudel, T.M., Tyron, W.W., and Purdum, C.M. (1998). Awareness of Disability and Long-Term Outcome After Traumatic Brain Injury. *Rehabilitation Psychology, 43*(4):267-281.

Varney, N.R. and Menefee, L. (1993). Psychosocial and Executive Deficits Following Closed Head Injury: Implications for Orbital Frontal Cortex. *Journal of Head Trauma Rehabilitation, 8*(1):32-44.

Wehman, P.H., West, M.D., Kregel, J., Sherron, P., and Kreutzer, J.S. (1995). Return to Work for Persons with Severe Traumatic Brain Injury: A Data-Based Approach to Program Development. *Journal of Head Trauma Rehabilitation, 10*(1):27-39.

Williams, W.H., Evans, J.J., Wilson, B.A., and Needham, P. (2002). Brief Report: Prevalence of Post-Traumatic Stress Disorder Symptoms After Severe Traumatic Brain Injury in a Representative Community Sample. *Brain Injury, 16*(8):673-679.

Chapter 2

Horticulture Therapy in the Treatment of Brain Injury

Ann Wedel
Gregory J. Murrey

INTRODUCTION AND OVERVIEW

Horticulture therapy is a complementary therapy or treatment modality that helps people to grow healthier in mind, body, and spirit using the natural connections between humans and nature. One can use houseplants, gardening, landscaping, and the natural world to improve the social, psychological, cognitive, and general health of their patients (Simson and Straus, 1998). Human beings are intricately connected to their environments and to the natural world. Ultimately people use horticulture therapy because they understand that gardens and the natural world uplift and benefit people (Lewis, 2000).

One can use the beauty of nature to heal suffering minds, bodies, and spirits by creating a sacred space and contemplative sanctuaries for individuals to just be themselves (Lewis, 2000). Horticulture therapy is based on the belief that nature heals and restores the longing soul. Nature speaks to people in a language that is perceived through their senses, and it gives them an opportunity to see how they fit into the larger design and complex tapestry of life (Lewis, 2000). A walk in the woods can be restoring, or working in a garden can be relaxing and uplifting. Nature is a modality that connects a person to his or her thoughts, emotions, and feelings (Lewis, 2000). Plants, gardens, and the natural world are used as conduits of healing and restoration.

The Use of Horticulture Therapy
with Medical Patients

It is common practice to bring plants or flowers to ailing and hospitalized loved ones. People intuitively know that a connection with nature is innately uplifting and healing. A growing body of research demonstrates the healing effects of nature with people who are recovering from serious illness. It has been found that just looking at pictures of nature or looking through a window into nature enhanced patients' ability to recuperate faster after surgery or serious illness. It was found that patients who were either actively or passively involved in nature used less pain medication, were able to get up and move about the room and facility more rapidly, and were discharged earlier than those who looked out of their windows into parking lots or at adjoining brick buildings and walls. Scenes of nature lower a person's stress response, causing positive physiological responses such as the lowering of irregularly high blood pressure and the reduction in muscle tension (Ulrich, 2000). It has a very powerful healing effect.

Horticulture therapists are trained professionals who understand the healing effect between a patient and the natural world and use it as a modality for support, restoration, and rehabilitation. Horticulture therapy has been used effectively for years in treating stroke, spinal cord injury, physical disabilities, developmental disabilities, mental illness, and for those suffering from substance abuse, the elderly as they are weakened by age, and even for the rehabilitation of prisoners (Simson and Straus, 1998).

The Use of Horticulture Therapy with Traumatically
Brain-Injured Patients

The business and commercialization of the modern world causes most people to suffer from wounds of isolation and invisibility. One of the most earnest needs of any human is to belong. One of the greatest pains any patient can have is a feeling of isolation and loneliness (Malidoma, 1999). Many who have suffered from a brain injury may incur a reduced sense of self and poor ego strength. They may have never been a part of a well-structured extended family nor ever known their place in this world. To be healthy, people need roots and to know they belong in this world. This grounding strength may never have been part of the TBI (traumatic brain injury) survivor's history, and thus they may need to work on healing the deep wounds of disconnection by connecting to spirit, community, and nature (Malidoma, 1999). Nature helps restore their well-being by easing their daily tensions and relieving their feelings of disconnection. By addressing their relationship with the visible worlds of nature and community, the individual can be healed (Malidoma, 1999).

Community is important because there is an understanding that human beings are collectively oriented. The general health and well-being of any individual is connected to a community. One's health and well-being is something that cannot be maintained alone or in a vacuum; however, people in the modern world are struggling with this. The pain from isolation and the stress of hyperstimulations brought on by the loss of community occurs for all of the human family (Malidoma, 1999). Following brain injury, isolation can become even more intense since the injured may find it harder to nurture themselves and their relationships with their families and friends. A necessity exists to help them heal through their natural connection to nature, which will help restore their feelings of belonging. Being part of a community will address the loneliness that plagues modern humankind (Malidoma, 1999).

Giving is the modus operandi for creating community and establishing a sense of belonging (Malidoma, 1999). Horticulture therapy is a medium in which people learn how to give again. A natural reciprocity is present in working with plants and the natural world; the more one gives the more one gets back. This learning to give and work with nature can be the beginning for patients to start restoring their diminishment and disconnection.

Community exists in part to safeguard the purpose of each person within it and to awaken the memory of that purpose by recognizing the unique gifts each individual brings to this world. People crave two things: to fully realize their innate gifts and to have these gifts approved, acknowledged, and confirmed. One's own confirmation or acknowledgment of themselves is not enough. The need to be acknowledged by others and society is utterly primal. People need restoration of community to fulfill to this deepest need (Malidoma, 1999).

Spirituality is about purpose, meaning, and being connected. It is about being connected to one's authentic self, with others, and with the world beyond (Lewis, 2000). However, one can be connected to their purpose only through the people around them (Malidoma, 1999). People can connect to their own spiritual wisdom when they are able to live and act as their authentic selves within their community. Healing comes when the individual remembers his or her identity and purpose. Human beings long for connection, and their sense of usefulness is derived from the feeling of connectedness (Malidoma, 1999).

Nature refreshes one's mind and spirit. Nature binds human beings to their beginnings and reconnects them with their own place in their own world. Nature provides calming, restoration, peacefulness, renewal, and refreshment to the mind and soul (Lewis, 2000). It enhances patients' ability to care for themselves as they learn to care for something outside of themselves. It helps people move toward nurturing not only themselves but also others. It helps them build relationships and community. Working with plants lessens one's intent to destroy and enhances the ability to assist in the creation of beauty and sanctuary. It helps raise self-esteem and confidence.

People have been dependent on the natural world and plants since the beginning of time (Lewis, 2000). Every tree, plant, hill, mountain, ocean, lake, river, and rock emanates at a subtle energy that has healing power, so if something in a person must change or heal, spending time in nature provides a good beginning (Malidoma, 1999). The natural world has provided inspiration, food, shelter, clothing, and medicine throughout the ages. A person's relationship to the natural world and to natural laws determined whether or not he or she lived or would be healed. Nature is the foundation of life and healing. Nature is a textbook for those who care to study it and a storehouse of remedies for all human ills. It is people's inborn ability to relate to nature that has let humanity evolve as it has (see Photo 2.1).

Being in nature opens the gates to deeper personal understanding and a sense of connectedness with the larger forces of the universe. One can consciously use this beautiful form of treatment through horticulture therapy to assist their patients in the restoration of their lives.

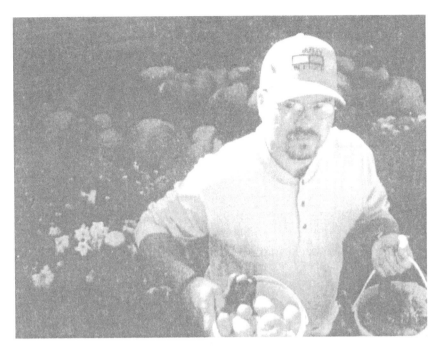

PHOTO 2.1. Patients may be more motivated to learn healthier eating habits when they grow and harvest their own produce. Reprinted with permission.

Goals of Horticulture Therapy with Brain Injury Patients

The goals of horticultural therapy with brain-injured patients should be:

- To provide patients access to a sanctuary of beauty and peace to decrease stress, anger, agitation, aggressive behavior, and anxiety while promoting comfort, nurturing, spiritual healing, and reflection.
- To provide patients with a setting for emotional and behavioral management, eliminating chemical dependency, and for psychological healing. Patients will have opportunities to experience joy and contentment. Staff should understand and promote a passive appreciation of just being in nature, knowing that pas-

sive appreciation is healing and can be just as effective as active participation. Staff should encourage the patients to find solace in nature and use natural calming environments to help them learn behavioral and emotional regulation skills.

- To create an aesthetic, beautiful healing space and environment in which a sense of personal space and a feeling of control exists for patients. Staff should encourage and help patients construct their own healing area. Patients should be encouraged to plant and maintain their own gardens.
- To help patients learn to nurture themselves and others by first learning to nurture plants and the environment. Staff should enhance patients' appreciation of their environment through horticulture therapy. Staff will help the patient develop an understanding of the impact of their actions on themselves, others, and their environment.
- To utilize organic gardening practices to minimize patients' contact with toxic substances. Staff should use horticulture therapy to teach patients to be good stewards of the earth as well as of themselves.
- To promote hope and improve self-efficacy. Staff should use nature and plants to help patients develop pride and accomplishment in achieving their goals. Horticulture therapy can be used to help promote self-esteem, independence, and self-confidence; it can champion creativity and self-expression; it can promote patient involvement and participation in meaningful tasks; and it can be used to increase self-initiated meaningful activities and provide opportunities for patients' achievement and success.
- To assist patients in developing a sense of personal responsibility and how to act in a more responsible fashion.
- To provide patients the opportunity to give back and be a contributing member of a community. It can help promote community involvement and integration. Horticulture therapy encourages patients to move away from egocentricity and into a mode of mutual sharing and giving so they can become aware of their impact on themselves and others. Participating in nature encourages patients to encourage others to participate in nature as well; they help others find hope as they help themselves. This therapy can

promote community through giving plants and produce away to those who would benefit from their contribution.

- To help patients select meaningful personalized learning goals. Horticulture therapy can be used to enhance patients' cognitive skills through working with plants and nature. It will be used to facilitate learning and to increase patients' attention to task, foresight, decision making, passage of time, and planning.
- To assist patients in establishing leisure-time skills that can fill voids once filled by less healthy activities. It can promote life-long recreational and vocational skills.
- To assist patients in building work ethics and skills through working with nature. It can be used to help develop or enhance prevocational and vocational skills.
- To assist patients in enhancing body awareness and effectiveness by helping patients develop physically through the enhancement of strength, mobility, endurance, coordination, and fine motor skills. The facility should provide for proper tools, appropriate pathways, and work surfaces so patients of differing physical abilities can complete their projects safely.
- To help staff evaluate progress based on the degree to which socialization occurs during the therapy, the extent to which resources were used, the extent to which patients perceived the activity as enjoyable and relaxing, and the extent to which patients assumed responsibility for the care of their plants, gardens, and tools.
- To ensure patients receive more individualized treatment through the use of trained staff and an ample and effective volunteer program.

HORTICULTURAL THERAPY GOALS FOR NEUROBEHAVIORALLY DISORDERED PATIENTS

The primary horticultural therapy service goals for individuals with TBI and related neurobehavioral disorders include the following:

- Reducing levels of agitation and aggressive behaviors
- Increasing self-initiated meaningful activity

- Facilitating physical, occupational, and other rehabilitation therapies in a nonconfrontational manner and in a natural setting
- Developing prevocational and vocational skills

Reduction of Agitation and Aggressive Behaviors

A naturally calming or emotionally relaxing activity for a TBI patient can be simply being outside of the hospital walls in a flourishing garden he or she helped create. Such an environment provides the patient with his or her own physical space and fewer stimuli than exists within the facility, or with at least more natural, calming stimuli. During horticultural therapy, staff can promote patient awareness of reduced body tension and a more calm emotional state while they are involved in the various activities. For example, rehabilitation staff from various disciplines can use this time with the patient to discuss issues and concepts related to aggression and behavioral dysfunction. Addressing reduction of agitation and aggressive behaviors becomes a primary treatment focus for clinicians working with such neurobehaviorally disordered patients (Sohlberg, Mateer, and Stuss, 1993; Trudel, Tyron, and Purdum, 1998; Grace, Stout, and Malloy, 1999; Prigatano, 1999). Thus, therapeutic approaches during horticultural therapy can include the application of physical and emotional control techniques during naturally and physically relaxing activities (Goldstein and Levin, 1995; Prigatano, 1999), methods of increasing anger and frustration thresholds (Hart and Jacobs, 1993; Sohlberg, Mateer, and Stuss, 1993; Varney and Menefee, 1993), and generalizing of various stress coping strategies. Such concepts and therapeutic interactions can occur on both an informal and formal basis. The horticultural therapy milieu, therefore, becomes a catalyst for staff and patients to address significant behavioral difficulties in a natural and nonthreatening environment.

Self-Initiated Meaningful Activity

Perhaps one of the most devastating consequences of severe brain injury is the patient's reduction in or total loss of meaningful activity in his or her life (Lezak, 1993), often resulting in clinical depression and/or exacerbation of agitation and inappropriate behavior. The lack of meaningful activity can be a direct result of the patient's neurologically based inability to initiate goal-directed behaviors. In addition, inappropriate social behavior such as impulsivity and physical aggression can be a primary barrier to participating in meaningful activities. Through horticultural therapy, the patient is given an opportunity to learn and participate in a routine, purposeful, goal-directed activity while introducing the complexity of cognitive demands slowly over time. Thus, within this safe and naturalistic environment, the patient is able to learn and apply self-initiation and self-regulation (social-behavioral) skills. For example, the patient may be coached on simple horticultural activities, such as following a watering schedule for plants in the greenhouse. Staff prompting to complete such simple tasks can then be slowly withdrawn or reduced. Additional activities such as weeding, planting, and planning a garden can be introduced to encourage patient responsibility for initiating/completing such activities with minimal staff assistance or prompting. Also, as horticultural activities can range from very basic to complex (both cognitively and physically), specific tasks can be introduced according to the patient's abilities and needs (see Photo 2.2).

Physical, Occupational, and Other Rehabilitation Therapy Goals

Because many patients with neurobehavioral disorders are often resistant to participating in rehabilitation therapies provided through traditional modalities (such as physical and occupational therapy), horticultural therapy staff can provide an environment conducive to positive, nonconfrontational, therapist-patient interaction. Patients tend to be in a more relaxed and nondefensive physical and mental state during the horticultural activities, thus therapists from various disciplines (including physical, occupational, rehabilitation nursing, behavioral, psychological, spiritual, and chemical dependency therapy) can use this time to work with patients on discipline-specific goals and treatments. For example, the physical therapist can work on activities to promote improved ambulation and mobility with the mutual goal of improving the patient's physical stamina so as to better care for his or her garden plot. The physical therapist can then incrementally increase the physical demands on the patient. Likewise, the behavioral therapist and psychologist can informally discuss with the patient how anger and aggression can be better con-

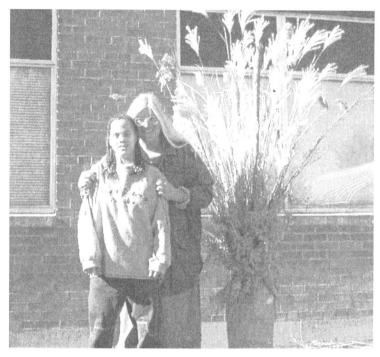

PHOTO 2.2. Floral design is a favorite activity for many patients in horticultural therapy. Such activity is used to promote creativity and improve cognitive planning skills. Reprinted with permission.

trolled by learning how to reduce body tension even during physical activity (see Photo 2.3).

Prevocational and Vocational Skills Training

Another devastating consequence of severe brain injury is a person's inability to return to gainful employment. As much of a person's self-image and self-esteem is determined by a person's occupation, the loss of vocational skills and ability due to cognitive, physical, and behavioral deficits can be catastrophic to the individual's emotional state and well-being. Unfortunately, the loss of involvement in vocational and even leisure activity exacerbates the emotional and behavioral disturbances. Through horticultural therapy, prevocational skill building and assessment can be conducted in a more emotionally and physically safe environment (as compared to a higher-stimuli, less-supervised

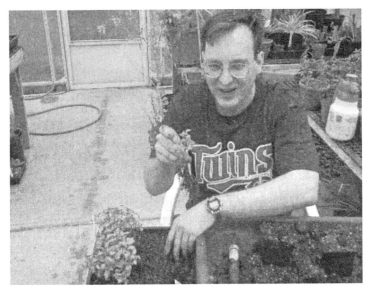

PHOTO 2.3. Here a patient is diligently using fine motor skills to transplant small seedlings in the greenhouse for later summer planting for his own garden. Reprinted with permission.

community setting). Also, during the horticultural therapy activity, the interdisciplinary team members can assist patients in regaining skills in cognitive (planning, problem solving, sequencing, attention, concentration, and mental flexibility), emotional/psychological (anger management, emotion regulation, and anxiety reduction), and physical abilities. For example, a patient may be given the responsibility to plan the layout of a garden or a section of the greenhouse and/or to develop activity and work schedules to maintain those areas. Such responsibilities are developed with the patient's individual abilities and needs in mind. In addition, staff may work with patients in learning and applying stress-reduction and frustration-tolerance techniques during the horticultural therapy activities.

REHABILITATION-HOSPITAL-BASED MODEL FOR A HORTICULTURAL THERAPY PROGRAM

The physical, logistical, and technical aspects of a hospital-based horticultural therapy program are typically carried out by a core horticultural staff, which includes physical, occupational, recreational, and horticultural therapy professionals. However, as previously discussed, the horticultural therapy program should be part of a holistic model, and therefore staff from all other disciplines in the hospital (behavioral therapy, nursing, pastoral care, rehabilitation psychology, etc.) should be actively involved in this therapeutic program. Staff from these various disciplines can provide informal individual and small-group therapeutic services as part of the horticultural therapy activity. The horticultural therapy staff should create a naturalistic, nonthreatening, and relaxed environment to promote positive, nonconfrontational interactions between patients and staff and to increase potential for patient participation in skills acquisition.

Physical Layout

The physical layout of a horticultural therapy program can include four primary features:

1. Seasonal vegetable, flower, and herb gardens
2. Hospital grounds landscaping area
3. Seasonal greenhouse
4. Hospital unit and patient room therapeutic areas

Seasonal Vegetable, Flower, and Herb Gardens

From early spring until mid-fall, the patients can become involved in outdoor horticultural programming helping to create gardens. The gardens should be designed to involve all of the senses. The sounds of the birds and the wind through trees in this natural setting enhance relaxation, attention, and listening skills. In addition, many herbs, plants, and fragrant flowers can be planted that positively stimulate the olfactory senses. The garden may also have a variety of fruit trees and vegetable plants that engage the sense of purposeful work since patients are involved in creating food for their own tables and to share with their families. In this manner patients can continuously work to create more visual beauty and to create a sense of personal space through the variation in textures, colors, hues, shapes, and forms.

Hospital Grounds Landscaping Area

The hospital grounds or atrium area provides an excellent opportunity for horticultural therapy. Many areas on the grounds can be converted into a therapeutic sanctuary. Staff and patients improve the grounds by designing and developing gardens to enhance healing, natural beauty, learning, and a stress-free environment.

Seasonal Greenhouse

Development of a small greenhouse can add a significant component to the horticultural therapy program. This is especially useful in regions with colder winter climates. State and federal grants are often available for development of therapeutic programs and might be obtained for such a project or service. Involving college students from a nearby college or university that has a horticultural or landscape design program is another helpful option. College students could work with staff and patients as volunteers or for college credits in designing and constructing the greenhouse or other horticultural therapy areas. Winter programming, with or without a greenhouse, can include patient instruction and training in all types of horticultural subjects, including propagation, transplanting, labeling, floral designing, pest control, soil analysis, proper watering, and care of plants. Student and staff involvement also provides patients the opportunity to interact with the community in a safe, structured, yet natural and real-life setting.

Hospital Unit and Patient Rooms

Each patient should be encouraged to bring plants into his or her living area and learn to care for them. In addition, fresh flowers can be brought into the hospital unit so that patients can make bouquets to keep in their private rooms. Patients can also be encouraged to share their plants with loved ones and with staff with whom they have developed a special relationship.

Patients' injuries are often so severe and the consequences so devastating that they may not be able to see beyond themselves. For some patients, the individualized horticultural therapy programming provides, for the first time since their injury, an opportunity to nurture something outside of themselves. The plants become their connection back to a world that includes something dependent upon them for care. The therapy also provides the opportunity to develop creativity and self-worth as well as increased control over their environment. This individualized component of horticultural therapy provides a wonderful, direct feedback loop for the patients on their own success, growth, and progress. Success of such programs are due in part to involvement by the local community. Donations of plants, cut flowers, and soil amendments made by local greenhouses, learning centers, farmers, floral shops, and garden stores can be sought as a means to enhance hospital-based horticultural programs and help ensure its success.

Horticultural Therapy Activities Schedule

Formal Horticultural Therapy Group

Formal horticultural therapy groups for patients can be provided at least two times per week under the coordination of the primary horticultural therapy staff. During this time, core horticultural staff conduct formal horticultural programming, training, education, and therapy on a variety of topics (gardening, plant care, greenhouse maintenance, etc.). Staff from other disciplines can also provide individual and small-group, discipline-specific therapeutic intervention and treatments. This training is conducted in one or more of the horticultural therapy sites depending on season, weather, and program needs.

Informal Individual or Small-Group Horticultural Therapies

Scheduled ad hoc therapeutic horticultural activities should be conducted with select patients throughout the week (including weekends and holidays). Staff trained in horticultural programming as well as in behavioral and recreational services typically conduct these services with the patients. These individual and small-group therapies typically occur five to seven days per week and at least one time per day. During these informal therapy sessions, patients have the opportunity to use and build upon their horticultural skills as well as to work on general rehabilitation and behavioral goals.

Special Horticultural Therapy Outings and Educational Field Trips

Several trips to the local arboretum, nature center, or even botanical gardens and parks can be scheduled for patients and staff. Throughout the year, such outings can provide patients and staff with a better understanding of horticultural program potentials and general educational opportunities to learn more about the horticultural process and the healing such environments can provide.

APPENDIX:
HORTICULTURAL THERAPY RESOURCES
AND CONTACT INFORMATION

Professional Certification and Organizations/Horticulture Resources and Contact Information

The American Horticulture Therapy Association
3570 E 12th Ave.
Denver, Colorado 80206
303-322-2482
www.ahta.org

Beverly Farm Foundation
6301 Humbert Rd.
Godfrey, Illinois 62035
618-466-0367
www.beverlyfarm.org

Bryn Mawr Rehab
413 Paoli Pike
Malvern, Pennsylvania 19355
610-251-5400
www.mcinlinehealth.org/br

The Canadian Horticulture Therapy Association
100 Westmount Rd.
Guelph, ON CANADA NIH 5H8
519-822-9842
www.chta.ca/about_us.

Carrier Foundation
County Rd. 601, PO Box 147
Belle Mead, New Jersey 08502
908-281-1000 Ext. 1222

Casa Colina Horticulture Therapy and Training Program
2801 N Garey Ave., PO Box 6001
Pomona, California 91760-6001
800-962-5462

Chicago Botanic Garden
PO Box 400
Glencoe, Illinois 60022
708-835-8300

Cleveland Botanical Garden
11030 East Blvd.
Cleveland, Ohio 44106
216-721-1600

Coler-Goldwater Specialty Hospital and Nursing Facility
1 Main St. Roosevelt Island
New York, New York 10044
212-318-8000

Colmery-O'Neil VA Medical Center
2200 Gage Blvd. (116B)
Topeka, Kansas 66622
785-350-3111

Delaware Center for Horticulture
1810 N Dupont St.
Wilmington, Delaware 19806
302-658-6282

Denver Botanic Garden
909 York St.
Denver, Colorado 80206
303-370-8040

Father Flanagan's Boys' Home
Horticulture Training Center
Boystown, Nebraska 68010
402-498-1100

The Federation to Promote Horticulture for Disabled People
The Geoffrey Udall Building
Trunkwell Park, Beech Hill Reading, England RG7 AT
www.cityfarmer.org/horttherp

Friends Hospital
4641 Roosevelt Blvd.
Philadelphia, Pennsylvania 19124
215-831-4600

Glass Garden/Rusk Institute of Rehabilitation Medicine
400 E 34th St.
New York, New York 10016
212-263-6058

The Holden Arboretum
9500 Sperry Rd.
Kirtland, Ohio 44060
216-256-1110 or 216-946-4400

Legacy Extended Care
1015 NW 22nd Ave. SE
Portland, Oregon 97210
503-413-6507

The Menninger Clinic
2801 Gessner Dr.
PO Box 809045
Houston, Texas 77280
800-351-9058

Minnesota Neurorehabilitation Hospital
11615 State Ave.
Brainerd, Minnesota 56401
218-828-6130 or 218-828-6123

Northwest Georgia Regional Hospital
1305 Redmond Circle
Rome, Georgia 30165-1307
706-295-6079 or 706-295-6709

Ozanam Home for Boys
412 E 137th St.
Kansas City, Missouri 64145
816-942-5600

Tangram Rehabilitation Network
5315 Nursery Rd.
Maxwell, Texas 78656
512-396-0667

Campus-Based Programs: Universities and Colleges Currently Offering Horticulture Therapy Programs or Courses

Denver Botanic Gardens
909 York St.
Denver, Colorado 80206-3799
303-370-8190

Edmonds Community College
20000 68th Ave. West
Lynnwood, Washington 98036
425-640-1459

Kansas State University
2021 Throckmorton Plant Sciences Center
Manhattan, Kansas 66506-5506
785-532-1420

Horticulture Therapy Elective Courses

Arizona State University
PO Box 871601
Tempe, Arizona 85287-1601
602-965-7735

College of DuPage
22nd St. and Lambert Rd.
Glen Ellyn, Illinois 60137-6599
630-942-3789

Horticulture Therapy Institute
PO Box 461189
Denver, Colorado 80246
303-388-0500

Metropolitan Community College
PO Box 3777
Omaha, Nebraska 68103
402-457-2309

Oklahoma State University
400 N Portland Ave.
Oklahoma City, Oklahoma 73107
405-947-4421 or 800-560-4099

Randolph Community College
PO Box 1009
Asheboro, North Carolina 27204
336-633-0235

Rockland Community College
145 College Rd.
Suffern, New York 10901
914-574-4273

SUNY Cobleskill
Agriculture and Natural Resources Division
Curtis Mott 100
Cobleskill, New York 12043-9986
518-255-5648

Temple University
Ambler, Pennsylvania 19002
215-283-1497

Tennessee Technical University
School of Agriculture
Box 5034
Cookeville, Tennessee 38505
615-372-3288

Tulsa Junior College
3727 East Apache
Tulsa, Oklahoma 74115
918-631-7566

University of Massachusetts
Durfee Conservatory
Amherst, Massachusetts 01002
413-545-5234

Certificate Programs

The New York Botanical Gardens
200th St. and S Boulevard
Bronx, New York 10458-5126
718-817-8747

Northern Virginia Community College
1000 Harry Flood Byrd Highway
Sterling, Virginia 20164-8699
703-450-2550

Distance Learning/Correspondence Course

Kansas State University
231-College Court Building
Manhattan, Kansas 66406-6007
913-532-5686

Horticultural-Therapy-Related Books and Resources

Kathleen Yeomans (1992). *The Able Gardener: Overcoming Barriers of Age and Physical Limitations.* Pownal, VT: Storey Communications.

Peter Please (Ed.). (1990). *Able to Garden: A Practical Guide for Disabled and Elderly Gardeners.* Charlotte, VT: Garden Way Publishing.

Janeen Adil (1993). *Accessible Gardening for People with Physical Disabilities: A Guide to Methods, Tools, and Plants.* Bethesda, WA: Idyll Arbor.

Philip Evans and Brian Donnelly (1993). *Accessible Landscapes: Designing for Inclusion.* San Francisco: SFSU Foundation Accessible Landscape Project.

Frank Schweller (1989). *Container Gardening for the Handicapped.* Phoenix: Hand-D-Cap Publishing.

Marilyn Barrett (1992). *Creating Eden: The Garden As a Healing Space.* San Francisco: Harper.

Gene Rothert (no date). *The Enabling Garden: Creating Barrier-Free Gardens.* Dallas: Taylor Publishing Co.

Jeffrey Restuccio (1992). *Fitness the Dynamic Gardening Way: A Health and Wellness Lifestyle.* Cordo, TN: Balance of Nature Publishing.

Lyn Dennis (1994). *Garden for Life: Horticulture for People with Special Needs.* Saskatoon SK Canada: University of Extension Press.

D. Hollinrake (1992). *Gardening: Equipment for Disabled People.* Oxford, UK: The Disability Information Trust.

Audrey Cloet and Chris Underhill (1990). *Gardening Is for Everyone.* London: Batsford Ltd.

Hans Schuman (no date). *Gardening Within Arm's Reach: Gardening and Experiencing Nature for the Visually Handicapped. How to Set Up a Garden with This in Mind.* The Netherlands: Bortimeus Utrechsewey.

Hank Bruce (1999). *Gardens for the Senses, Gardening As Therapy.* Winter Spring, FL: Winner Enterprises.

Clare Cooper Marcus and Marni Barnes (1995). *Gardens in Health Care Facilities: Uses, Therapeutic Benefits and Design Recommended.* Berkeley, CA: The Center for Health Design.

Charles Lewis (no date). *Green Nature/Human Nature: The Meaning of Plants in Our Lives.* Albuquerque, NM: People Plant Interaction.

Bobby Moore (1989). *Growing with Gardening: A Twelve Month Guide for Therapy, Recreation, and Education.* Chapel Hill, NC: University of North Carolina Press.

Mark Francis, Patricia Lindsey, and Jay Stone Rice (1994). *Healing Dimensions of People-Plant Relations.* Blacksburg, VA: Office of Environmental Horticulture.

Mitchell Hewson (1995). *Horticulture As Therapy: A Practical Guide to Using Horticulture As a Therapeutic Tool.* Guelph, Ontario, Canada: Homewood Health Center.

E. Matuso and P.D. Relf (1997). *Horticulture in Human Life, Culture, and Environment.* Koto, Japan: Aota Horticulturae.

Suzanne Wells (1997). *Horticultural Therapy and the Older Adult Population.* Binghamton, NY: The Haworth Press.

Jane Stoneham and Peter Thoday (1994). *Landscape Design for Elderly and Disabled People.* Wappingers Falls, NY: Garden Art Press.

Lynda Lloyd Nebbe (1991). *Nature As a Guide.* Minneapolis: Educational Medic Corp.

Joel Flagler and Raymond P. Pinelot (1994). *People-Plant Relationships: Setting Research Priorities.* Blacksburg, VA: People Plant Council.

N. Allan (1993). *A Personal Philosophy and Practical Approach to Horticulture Therapy.* Waverly, Australia: Embassy Press.

Diane Relf (Ed.) (1992). *The Role of Horticulture in Human Well-Being and Social Development.* Blacksburg, VA: Timber Press.

REFERENCES

Goldstein, R.C. and Levin, H.S. (1995). Neurobehavioral Outcome of Traumatic Brain Injury: Coma, the Vegetative State, and the Minimally Responsive State. *Journal of Head Trauma Rehabilitation, 10*(1): 57-73.

Grace, J., Stout, J.C., and Malloy, P.F. (1999). Assessing Frontal Lobe Behavioral Syndromes with the Frontal Lobe Personality Scale. *Psychological Assessment Resources, 6*(3): 269-284.

Hart, T. and Jacobs, H.E. (1993). Rehabilitation and Management of Behavioral Disturbances Following Frontal Lobe Injury. *Journal of Head Trauma Rehabilitation, 8*(1): 1-12.

Lewis, Charles A. (2000). The Evolutionary Importance of People-Plant Relationships. Presented at Minnesota Landscape Arboretum Conference, November 2, 2000: 11.

Lezak, M.D. (1993). Newer Contributions to the Neuropsychological Assessment of Executive Functions. *Journal of Head Trauma Rehabilitation, 8*(1): 24-31.

Malidoma, Patrice Some (1999). *The Healing Wisdom of Africa: Finding Life Purpose Through Nature, Ritual, and Community.* New York: Putnam, Inc.

Prigatano, G.P. (1999). *Principles of Neuropsychological Rehabilitation.* London: Oxford University Press.

Simson, Sharon and Straus, Martha (1998). *Horticulture As Therapy: Principles and Practice.* Binghamton, NY: The Haworth Press.

Sohlberg, M.M., Mateer, C.A., and Stuss, D.T. (1993). Contemporary Approaches to the Management of Executive Control Dysfunction. *Journal of Head Trauma Rehabilitation, 8*(1): 45-58.

Trudel, T.M., Tyron, W.W., and Purdum, C.M. (1998). Awareness of Disability and Long-Term Outcome After Traumatic Brain Injury. *Rehabilitation Psychology, 43*(4): 267-281.

Ulrich, Roger S. (2000). Evidence-Based Garden Design for Improving Health Outcomes. Presented at Minnesota Landscape Arboretum Conference, November 2, 2000: 30.

Varney, N.R. and Menefee, L. (1993). Psychosocial and Executive Deficits Following Closed Head Injury: Implications for Orbital Frontal Cortex. *Journal of Head Trauma Rehabilitation, 8*(1): 32-44.

Chapter 3

Art As a Therapeutic Modality with TBI Populations

Mark Sell
Gregory J. Murrey

INTRODUCTION AND OVERVIEW

According to the American Art Therapy Association (AATA),

> Art therapy is the therapeutic use of art making, within a profes-
> sional relationship, by people who experience illness, trauma, or
> challenges in living, and by people who seek personal develop-
> ment. Through creating art and reflecting on the art products
> and processes, people can increase awareness of self and others,
> cope with symptoms, stress, and the traumatic experiences, en-
> hance cognitive abilities, and enjoy the life-affirming pleasures
> of making art. (AATA, 2002)

Thus, art therapy experience provides clients a way to facilitate
change in behavior or personality that can last beyond the therapy
session (Winner, 1982).

Art making is a nonverbal tool that can be used to enhance communication about emotional and internal conflicts. An art therapy session can offer a positive, less performance-based alternative to traditional talk therapies. The nonverbal aspect of art psychotherapy holds
an important and unique position in the realm of mental health work
since it gives the client an opportunity to listen with his or her eyes.
This is specifically significant in our current society in which we are
constantly bombarded by speech through personal contact and communication media. The common tendency of individuals to tune out

what they prefer not to hear makes visual images powerful tools for treatment (Landgarten, 1981). TBI (traumatic brain injury) clients often have less tolerance to structure, but through art therapies they can be provided the opportunity to express themselves in an environment that is more creative, less confrontational, and more individualized.

Many traditional therapies are often based on concrete expectations of progress and pressure to be discharged from an inpatient TBI program. Art therapies focus more on process than concrete, end goals.

Clients with TBI feel losses acutely, including the loss of control over their lives. The feelings of anger that accompany these losses become a very real component in the client's life. In addition, clients face loss of cognitive insight, which can result in the client feeling intimidated and becoming resistant to traditional therapeutic approaches. Art activities provide a less-structured, stress-reducing process that reinforces positive ways of expression that break down the resistance and barriers to successful therapy. Along with resistance, clients with TBI often bring a sense of what is "good" art and what is "bad" art to the session as well as qualifiers for each. Two major factors influencing how clients with TBI view art may be cessation of drawing or painting at an early age or a previous negative experience with art making. People of earlier generations (such as the Depression era) rarely had time for leisure pastimes and often regard such activity as merely "kindergarten stuff" (Fausek, 1997).

Although clients with TBI may approach art therapy guardedly, a therapist can employ several creative ways to offer the art process on a nonthreatening basis. For example, a therapist may label a session as "arts and crafts" to break through the initial resistance. Some typical negative responses to art making include "I hate art," "I can't make my hands work," or "I'll look stupid." Despite these arguments, a variety of approaches to "sell" art therapy may be used. If a client with TBI enjoys the creative process, the therapist or group leader can gradually introduce more controversial themes.

> Clients who are extremely resistant to treatment and refuse to talk about themselves or their problems tend to activate counter-transference in the therapist. It is the author's belief that many art psychotherapists have less difficulty with this type of indi-

vidual since the client (engaged in such an art task) is communicating on a symbolic level. It is this factor which often enables the art psychotherapist to remain interested in the silent or "defensive" client. (Landgarten, 1981)

Rapport with the therapist or group leader is important, especially when building a trust relationship. The trust earned may allow the therapist to open up and express traumatic history or allow a positive confrontation to a daily episode of maladaptive behavior.

The art therapy process can focus on specific issues such as behavior management difficulties that have been identified in the client's treatment plan. Patient interaction with the treatment team and observations of the patient in sessions adds a holistic dimension to a client's treatment. For example, one positive result of art therapy may be to help a client identify and control certain behaviors that are a result of the TBI. As art and other creative activities tend to be soothing, enjoyable, and relaxing, the patient may readily experience success in controlling such behaviors during the art therapy session.

Art therapy sessions for clients with TBI should be structured to create the least amount of confrontation and anxiety for the participant. Establishing ground rules before a session with a small group of perhaps three to four will improve the likelihood of success with the process. For example, a group leader can set the tone of a session by identifying several "rules" for the group. This outline for expected behavior by group participants should enforce the idea that art making is very personal and that scrutinizing another person's artwork would not be welcomed. Creating trusting relationships among the participants is as crucial as the trusting relationship between patient and therapists. In order to maintain trust in the therapeutic process, the group leader should ask the participants what information the therapist may share with other treatment team professionals.

The therapy session can provide a safe place for autonomous creation; when involved in an inpatient TBI program, it is essential to allow clients the opportunity to feel a sense of control over the process. During the initial art therapy sessions, the group leader lends clients his/her ego strength and guides the clients through the session process. Ideally, the need for an art therapist to carefully or directly guide sessions will fade as the independence and confidence of the patient increases. Some secondary benefits from participating in art therapy sessions include increased stamina and tolerance to various environmental barriers, increased dexterity and hand-eye coordination, improved initiation of sequential activities, increased on-task duration, and reduction of agitation. Art therapy is a subtle therapy and is best conducted in low-stimuli settings. Inasmuch as art is considered a traditional nonverbal form of communication, social growth encouraged by the art therapist balances the nonverbal representations with verbal elicited communication. Interaction with the art therapist and other group participants promotes social skills and ultimately self-understanding for the client with TBI (Winner, 1982).

ART THERAPY WITHIN A TBI REHABILITATION PROGRAM

Although a growing body of literature demonstrates the effectiveness of art therapy and other expressive arts with a variety of disability groups (Kramer, 1977; Ulman, 1975; DiCowden, 1987; Sourkes, 1991; Kingsley and Pfeuffer, 1982; Miller, 1998; Weaver, 2001; Canner Hume and Hitti, 1988), very little has been published on the role of art therapy for persons with severe traumatic brain injury (McGraw, 1989; Barker and Brunk, 1991; Lazarus-Leiff, 1998; Rosner, 2000). In particular, few to no recent publications describe in detail (1) the format and specific goals of an art therapy program for persons with traumatic brain injury and associated neurobehavioral and emotional disturbances, (2) special considerations of TBI clients' unique cognitive and behavioral dysfunction deficits and how these will affect an art therapy program, or (3) the interface between art therapy and rehabilitation psychology services. The purpose of this section is, therefore, to outline the goals, approaches, and structure of an inpatient therapeutic art program and how the individual TBI patient's neurobehavioral goals and issues are addressed. In addition, the interface between members of the rehabilitation team (including rehabilitation psychology) will be discussed.

Goals of Therapeutic Art for the Person with TBI

Through the therapeutic art program, four primary needs of the TBI patient (cognitive/emotional, psychological/spiritual, physical, and behavioral) are addressed as part of the holistic rehabilitation approach (see Figure 3.1 in color art section at end of chapter). The primary goals of the art therapy services for the traumatic brain-injured person should include the following:

- To increase self-initiated leisure and creative activity
- To provide an alternative modality for assessments to better understand the patient
- To promote expression of emotions and thoughts not often expressed in a socially appropriate manner
- To increase cognitive and physical (fine motor coordination) functioning
- To reduce levels of agitation and aggressive behaviors

As described in Chapter 2, persons with severe TBI often present with executive functioning deficits, which includes a diminished ability to initiate appropriate, goal-directed, meaningful activity. Perhaps one of the most devastating consequences of a TBI is the patient's reduction in or total loss of meaningful activity in his or her life. Such a loss can often lead to clinical depression (Rosenthal, Christensen, and Ross, 1998) and exacerbation of agitation and inappropriate behaviors. The lack of meaningful activity can be a direct result of the patient's neurologically based inability to initiate goal-directed behaviors (Lezak, 1993; Varney and Menefee, 1993; Prigatano, 1999). Thus, the patient's opportunity and ability to participate in leisure, fulfilling, and stress-reducing activities is significantly diminished. In addition, inappropriate social behavior such as impulsivity and physical aggression can be a primary barrier to participating in meaningful activities, including employment (Buffington and Malec, 1997). Through art therapies, the patient is able to learn and participate in such activities while slowly increasing the complexity of cognitive demands over time.

Increase Self-Initiated Leisure
and Creative Activity

Through the art therapy process, the TBI patient is able to increase self-initiation in an incremental or stepwise fashion. Since art therapy activities can be structured from simple to more complex tasks, the process can be tailored to the individual's specific needs and abilities. For example, for a patient with severe initiation dysfunction, a simple staff cuing system can be implemented early in the therapeutic process by setting the patient at a table, with a pencil or marker and piece of paper on the table. The staff then may provide a simple command to the patient such as "go ahead and draw something." Even for persons with significant initiation deficits or motor apraxia, visual and/or verbal cues will often elicit an initial automatic response such as reaching out and picking up the pencil. With subsequent sessions, patients are given increasingly more complex tasks or assignments with a goal of the patient initiating a creative task with few to no prompts.

An Alternative Modality for Assessment
to Better Understand the Patient

Art therapy techniques provide psychology and other rehabilitation staff additional information regarding the patient's psychological functioning. Projective techniques such as journaling, creative writing, and freehand drawing have long been used as psychological assessments and techniques. Such techniques help elicit information regarding the person's unconscious thoughts and beliefs by promoting freer expression of possible underlying psychopathology. Art therapy activities thus can provide a nonconfrontive and subtle modality to help the rehabilitation psychologist and other rehabilitation team members better understand the person, and his or her motivations and psychological functioning. Through structured assessment techniques, the art therapist, in coordination with the rehabilitation psychologist, can gain important insights regarding the patient's psychological constructs and motivation. Such information is then communicated to other rehabilitation team members (including the psychiatrist, chaplain, behavioral analyst, and chemical dependency counselor) to incorporate into individual and group therapy sessions.

Promoting Expression of Emotions and Thoughts
Often Not Previously Disclosed

A variety of cognitive, emotional, and behavioral deficits secondary to the brain injury can result in the patient experiencing a diminished ability to express emotions. For example, word fluency, word finding, and other expressive language disorders can be a direct result of the neurological trauma after brain injury. In addition, other neurocognitive and neurobehavioral deficits may impede the patient's ability to organize thoughts, formulate appropriate sentences, and regulate emotions during high-stress situations. The patient may also present with diminished ability or opportunity to participate in naturally stress-reducing activities. Art therapy activities, thus, can be a medium for enhancing emotional expression such as fear, anger, sadness, grief, and distress in a less anxiety-provoking situation. Although journaling and writing may be an additional form of expression, many TBI patients may have lost (or may never have had) the ability to express themselves through this modality. Thus, as agraphia and constructional apraxia are common postinjury, other expressive modalities provided through art therapies may be highly beneficial. Severe TBI can often result in a decreased ability to recognize one's own deficits, formally called *anosognosia*. Use of art therapy techniques can help promote insight even in persons presenting with severe agnosias. Continuous interactions and collaboration among the art therapist, psychologist, and chaplain provide for discussion of the issues and feelings revealed by patients during art therapy sessions.

Increase Cognitive and Physical (Fine Motor) Functioning

Many neurobehaviorally disordered TBI patients are resistant to participating in traditional rehabilitation therapies provided through traditional modalities (such as physical, occupational, and cognitive therapy). Art therapy activities provide an environment conducive to positive, nonconfrontational therapist/patient interaction. Patients tend to be in a more relaxed and nondefensive physical, mental, and emotional state during art therapy activities and thus are much more willing (even unknowingly so) to participate in activities that promote improvements in cognitive, psychomotor, and other physical functionings. For example, art therapy is a useful tool for enhancing learning and problem-solving abilities (Very Special Arts, 1993; Kingsley and Pfeuffer, 1982; Miller, 1998), which are common cognitive deficits and contributors to neurobehavioral dysfunction in persons with traumatic brain injury. Thus, in coordination with the physical and occupational therapists, neuropsychologist, and physicians, the art therapist can design and implement art therapy activities that directly address the discipline-specific goals. For a patient with psychomotor difficulties, for example, an individual plan can be designed that incrementally increases the difficulty of the task over each session. Also, art therapy activities can range from very basic to complex (both cognitively and physically), so specific therapies can be introduced according to the patient's individual abilities and needs. During daily patient rounds and weekly treatment planning meetings, the art therapist coordinates with the psychologist and the physical and occupational therapists to develop an art therapy treatment plan.

Reducing Agitation and Aggressive Behaviors

It is physically impossible for the body to experience relaxation/calmness and anxiety/agitation (arousal) at the same time (Jacobson, 1948; Jacobson, 1938; Wolpe, 1969). Art therapy activities provide TBI patients with an environment for naturally calming activities. During these activities, the art therapist promotes patient awareness of body tension and emotional state. The art therapist or psychologist may also use this time with the patient to discuss issues and concepts related to aggression, behavioral dysfunction, emotion regulation, and appropriate expression of negative emotions (Grace, Stout, and Malloy, 1999; Sohlberg, Mateer, and Stuss, 1993; Trudel, Tyron, and Purdum, 1998; Prigatano, 1999). Such conceptual discussions and therapeutic interactions occur on both an informal and formal basis. Thus, the art therapy milieu becomes a catalyst for staff and patients to address significant behavioral and emotional difficulties in a natural and nonthreatening environment.

HOSPITAL-BASED PROGRAMS

Initial Assessment and Participant Selection

Following the admission of a new inpatient at a hospital, an initial and comprehensive art and recreational therapy assessment is conducted. During the assessment process, an individual's needs, interests, and goals are identified. Via the assessment it is determined if the patient is appropriate for participation in the therapeutic art program. The art therapist then meets with a rehabilitation team during the initial treatment planning meeting to review the patient's cognitive, behavioral, emotional, and physical issues. Once the team and discipline-specific patient goals are identified, an art therapy plan is developed.

Art Therapy Process and Activities

The art therapist meets with inpatients on both an individual and group basis. In addition, individual patients may be given art therapy homework assignments to be completed during nontherapy time. The art therapy staff meet regularly with the rehabilitation team members to discuss the patient's progress and issues, and to plan revisions.

CASE EXAMPLES

Case #1: Another Evaluation

This thirty-seven-year-old female patient with a post-TBI history of self-injury, depression, and aggression was asked to express a reaction to a current disappointment and how she felt. This patient had a scheduled pass with her family but had a serious setback behaviorally. The team decided that due to demonstrated instability, the pass should be postponed. She drew a picture (Figure 3.1) representing her feelings after the team informed her of the canceled pass. The patient stated that frustration, panic, and loss of autonomy were shown in the drawing. She also commented on how she was trying to appear in control and to give a calmer appearance than what she was actually experiencing "inside."

Case #2: Disrespect

A patient was asked to express herself regarding an incident in which she was involved. The patient was a twenty-nine-year-old female of medium size who had engaged in a physical assault against a male who was six feet five inches tall and weighed approximately 325 pounds. The assault was severe in nature and, by her admission, was not well thought-out. Impulsive behavior is often a common result of a TBI injury, and the opportunity to reflect on it can be therapeutic in an artistic environment. Her artwork (Figure 3.2) symbolizes a runaway forest fire along with futile attempts by the staff to "cool off the situation." The cigarette in the left corner was the catalyst for the incident. She reflected that the patient had "insulted" her by intentionally flicking the cigarette butt in her direction and she reacted violently. She admitted that she exaggerated the gravity of this incident and caused a great deal of negative fallout, which she later regretted. Compensatory strategies for dealing with this type of conflict were introduced during this discussion.

Case #3: Drunk

In this case, a patient was given an assignment of re-creating a social or cultural period she could reflect on as either a positive or negative influence on her life. The patient was a twenty-seven-year-old female with a post-TBI history of chemical abuse and other impulse-control disorders. The patient's artwork is provided in Figure 3.3. In reference to her artwork, she stated that during her "partying days" she made huge mistakes that compromised her future and health, but that short-term euphoria and peer pressure often was greater than her better judgment. Discussion about chemical-dependency issues in the group resulted in an open and frank exchange on how chemical dependency is addressed in conjunction with traumatic brain injury and pharmacology strategies.

Case #4: Marooned

Family dynamics were the topic of this art therapy project assignment. The patient was a twenty-two-year-old male with a post-TBI history of physical aggression and inappropriate social interactions. The patient indicated a feeling of desertion by his family after his injury. The picture he drew is provided in Figure 3.4. He characterized the rocks as his rehabilitation treatment center and felt aground at this period. He said the fishing represented his attitude regarding his progress. He felt if he could achieve his "limit" he could be able to get "to shore." Impeding rough weather was symbolic of his anger that often would build in frustrating situations. He mentioned that birds were a symbol of hope because it meant land was somewhere within reach and he could regain more of his independence. He also indicated that his depiction of himself being in the middle of this water was indicative of how he felt surrounded by events that were out of his control.

Case #5: Conflicted

This art therapy activity was designed as a projective assessment measure. The patient was a forty-two-year-old female with a long history of drug abuse and post-TBI sexual impulsivity who was asked to draw what made her happy. In this particular case the patient had been involved in art therapy for approximately three weeks and had become fairly comfortable in freely initiating and participating in the therapeutic activity. The patient produced the drawing in Figure 3.5. Without any comment or discussion of this initial drawing, the patient was then asked to turn the paper over and to draw something else that made her happy. The patient then produced the drawing in Figure 3.6. In session with the art therapist and psychologist present, the patient was asked to discuss what she had drawn. When discussing the first drawing (Figure 3.5) the patient stated, "This is a picture of me with my husband walking the dog." She then discussed the second drawing stating, "This is me doing drugs. It is something that makes me happy." The patient then became quite tearful and clearly recognized the conflict (dissonance) between these two parts of her life. This patient had lost her family because of her chemical abuse, which began after her head injury. Due to the associative anosognosia, she was not able (up to that point) to clearly recognize the consequences of her impulsive behaviors. However, through the use of this art therapy technique, a therapeutic door was opened for more productive discussion with her therapist about her conflicting emotions and behaviors, which increased insight into these issues. The activity was also a very powerful therapeutic tool that promoted initial insight into self-defeating and inappropriate behaviors (especially when considering her lack of insight or agnosia).

Case #6: Season of Discontent

The theme of this exercise was an expression of family relations. This particular depiction by a twenty-eight-year-old TBI patient indicated a great deal of resentment and control issues with his father (see Figure 3.7). The color yellow was used to represent his outgoing attitude and general outlook on life; however, the color blue represented the issues of control and autonomy surrounding his postinjury relationship with his father over such circumstances as his new living situation and money dispensation, which resulted in constant conflict. As the patient discussed these conflicts he came to realize that a more objective approach to dealing with his father would be more helpful and successful.

Case #7: Split Personality

This case involved a thirty-seven-year-old female who had suffered a traumatic brain injury in a motor vehicle accident. The art therapy exercise was designed to be a conduit for self-expression about conflict in interpersonal relations with family and peers. Her explanation of her depiction (see Figure 3.8) of this particular lion was that it represented duality and internal conflict. She expressed that sometimes she felt she was being torn apart by something wild inside her. She indicated that the lion was the wild animal that could be unleashed at any time. She feared that this stronger, more dominant and aggressive side would overtake her personality and manifest itself in harmful behavior to both herself and others. Discussion with her psychologist about her interpretation of her drawing resulted in more effective treatment in this type of interconflict.

PATIENT OUTCOMES

Art therapy is only one component of an interdisciplinary, holistic rehabilitation program at a rehabilitation hospital. As such, it is difficult to fully evaluate the contribution of an art therapy program in isolation from other therapeutic services and programs. However, postdischarge behavioral evaluations and studies have shown promising findings since the formal introduction of art therapy programs at hospitals. Specifically, postdischarge outcome studies of patients in a three-year follow-up study suggest that patients maintain their behavioral stability and gains over time, with many still applying their skills, knowledge, and interests in recreational and expressive art activities in the community (Murrey et al., 2004). However, continued and more in-depth formal research on the benefits of art therapy with persons with traumatic brain injury and associated neurobehavioral disorders is needed.

TRAINING AND CERTIFICATION REQUIREMENTS

Professional training and board certification for art therapists is overseen by the American Art Therapy Association (AATA) and the Art Therapy Credentials Board (ATCB). The AATA regulates and oversees educational and professional ethical standards for trained/ certified art therapists. The current AATA educational requirements include the following:

- Master's degree in art therapy (or)
- Master's degree with an emphasis in art therapy (or)
- Twenty-four semester units in art therapy with a master's degree in a related field (or)
- Certification requirements to become a registered art therapist (ATR) (or)
- Board-certified art therapist (ATR-BC)

Qualifications as an ATR include the aforementioned educational requirements and completing a minimum of 1,000 direct client-contact hours under supervision. Additional requirements and qualifications are necessary for board certification. Persons interested in art therapy training or certification may wish to consult the AATA Web site at <www.arttherapy.org>.

APPENDIX: TRAINING AND ACADEMIC PROGRAMS

The following is a list of graduate-level education programs that have received approval from the AATA for a specific period of time, not exceeding seven years. The initial approval date is listed; therefore, those using this list should check the program's expiration date.

Adler School of Professional Psychology (initial approval 1999)
MA in Counseling Psychology: Art Therapy.
Contact: Judy Sutherland, PhD, ATR-BC, LCPC
Coordinator, Art Therapy Programs
65 East Wacker Place, Suite 2100
Chicago, Illinois 60601-7298
312-201-5900 Ext. 220
JHS@Adler.edu, <http://www.adler.edu>

College of New Rochelle (initial approval 1984)
MS in Art Therapy
Contact: Patricia St. John, EdD, ATR-BC
Program Coordinator, Graduate Art Therapy
29 Castle Place
New Rochelle, New York 10805-2339
914-654-5279 or 914-654-5280
pstjohn@cnr.edu, <http://www.cnr.edu>

Concordia University (initial approval 1987)
MA in Creative Art Therapies: Art Therapy and Drama Therapy Options
Contact: Josee Leclerc, PhD, ATR, ATPQ
1455 de Maisonneuve Boulevard West
Montreal, Quebec, Canada H3G 1M8
514-848-4683
Fax: 514-848-4790
cats@vax2.concordia.ca, <http://art-therapy.concordia.ca>

Drexel University College of Nursing and Health Professions
(initial approval 1979)
Health Sciences; MA in Art Therapy; Specialized Electives in Medical Art
    Therapy; Forensic Art Therapy; and Art Therapy in an Educational Setting

Contact: Nancy Gerber, PhD, ATR-BC, LPC
Director, Graduate Art Therapy Education
Hahnemann Center City Campus
1505 Race Street, Mail Stop 905
Philadelphia, Pennsylvania 19102-1192
215-762-6928 or 800-2-Drexel, Ext. 6333
Nancy.Gerber@drexel.edu, <http://cnhp.drexel.edu/GradProgs/Creative
   Arts/Art Therapy/>

Eastern Virginia Medical School (initial approval 1984)
MS in Art Therapy
Contact: Kay Stovall, ATR-BC
Graduate Art Therapy Program
PO Box 1980
Norfolk, Virginia 23501-1980
757-446-5895
artthrpy@evms.edu, <http://www.evms.edu/hlthprof/art-therapy.html>

Emporia State University (initial approval 1991)
MS in Art Therapy
Contact: Emily Endreson, MA, ATR-BC
Program Director, Art Therapy
1200 Commercial Street, Campus Box 4031
Emporia, Kansas 66801-5087
620-341-5809
endresoe@emporia.edu, <http://www.emporia.edu/psyspe/arttherapy/athp
   .html>

George Washington University (initial approval 1979)
MA Art Therapy
Contact: Anne Mills, MA, ATR-BC, LPC
Director, Art Therapy Program
2129 G Street NW, Building L, Rear
Washington, DC 20052
202-994-6285
amills@gwu.edu, <http://www.gwu.edu/~artx>

Hofstra University (initial approval 1984)
MA in Creative Arts Therapy, MS in Special Education: Art Therapy
Contact: Joan Bloomgarden, PhD, ATR-BC, CGP
Graduate Art Therapy Program
124 Hofstra University
Hempstead, New York 11549-1240

516-463-5300 or 516-463-5752
Joanbloomgarden@hofstra.edu, <http://www.hofstra.edu>

Lesley University (initial approval 1982)
MA in Expressive Therapies; MA in Art Therapy; and Mental Health
   Counseling Specialization
Contact: Susan Spaniol, ATR-BC
Coordinator of Art Therapy, Expressive Therapies Division
29 Everett Street
Cambridge, Massachusetts 02138
617-349-8436
sspaniol@mail.lesley.edu, <http://www.lesley.edu>

Long Island University, C.W. Post Campus (initial approval 1996)
MA in Clinical Art Therapy
Contact: Christine Kerr, PhD, ATR-BC, CGP
Director of Graduate and Undergraduate Clinical Arts Therapies
720 Northern Boulevard
Brookville, New York 11548
516-299-2935
christine.kerr@liu.edu, <http://www.liu.edu/~svpa/art>

Loyola Marymount University (initial approval 1979)
MA in Marital and Family Therapy
Contact: Debra Linesch, PhD, ATR-BC
Graduate Department of Marital and Family Therapy
One LMU Drive
Los Angeles, California 90045-2659
310-338-4562
lgloyd@lmu.edu, <http://www.lmu.edu/mft>

Marylhurst University (initial approval 1991)
MA in Art Therapy
Contact: Christine Turner, ATR-BC, LPC, NCC
Graduate Program in Art Therapy
17600 Pacific Highway (Hwy 43), PO Box 261
Marylhurst, Oregon 97036-0261
503-699-6244
cturner@marylhurst.edu or studentinfo@marylhurst.edu,
   <http://www.marylhurst.edu>

Marywood University (initial approval 1986)
MA in Art Therapy
Contact: Barbara Parker-Bell, MA, ATR-BC

Acting Director
2300 Adams Avenue
Scranton, Pennsylvania 18509-1598
570-348-6278 x 2525
parkerbell@es.marywood.edu, <http://www.marywood.edu>

Mount Mary College (initial approval 1995)
MS in Art Therapy
Contact: Bruce Moon, PhD, ATR-BC MA, MDiv
2900 North Menominee River Parkway
Milwaukee, Wisconsin 53222-4545
414-256-1215
moonb@mtmary.edu, <http://www.mtmary.edu>

Naropa University (initial approval 1998)
MA in Transpersonal Counseling Psychology: Concentration
    in Art Therapy
Contact: Michael Franklin, MA, ATR-BC, LSW
Program Director
2130 Arapaho Avenue
Boulder, Colorado 80302
800-772-6951
admissions@naropa.edu or michaelf@naropa.edu,
    <http://www.naropa.edu>

Nazareth College of Rochester (initial approval 1992)
MS in Art Therapy
Contact: Ellen G. Horovitz, PhD, ATR-BC
Director of Art Therapy
4245 East Avenue
Rochester, New York 14618-3790
585-389-2535
eghorovi@naz.edu, <http://www.naz.edu/dept/art_therapy/index.html>

New York University (initial approval 1979)
MA in Art Therapy
Contact: Ikuko Acosta, PhD, ATR-BC
Director of Graduate Art Therapy Program
34 Stuyvesant Street
New York, New York 10003
212-998-5726 or 212-998-5727
ia4@nyu.edu, <http://www.nyu.edu>

Notre Dame de Namur University (initial approval 1986)
MA in Art Therapy; MA in Marriage and Family Therapy
Contact: Doris Arrington, EdD, ATR-BC
Chair, Art Therapy Program
1500 Ralston Avenue
Belmont, California 94002
650-508-3556
Arttherapy@ndnu.edu, <http://www.ndnu.edu>

Phillips Graduate Institute (initial approval 2003)
MA in Psychology with a major in Marriage and Family
   Therapy/Art Therapy
Contact: Noah Hass-Cohen, MA, ATR-BC
Director of Art Therapy and Core Faculty
5445 Balboa Boulevard
Encino, California 91316-1509
818-386-5611
noah@pgi.edu, <http://www.laiat.com> <http://www.pgi.edu>

Pratt Institute (initial approval 1980)
MPS in Art Therapy and Creativity Development;
   MPS in Art Therapy: Special Education
Contact: Laurel Thompson, MPS, ADTR, ATR-BC
Chairperson, Graduate Creative Arts Therapy Department
East 3, 200 Willoughby Avenue
Brooklyn, New York 11205
718-636-3428
Lthompso@pratt.edu, <http://www.pratt.edu>

School of the Art Institute of Chicago (initial approval 1989)
MA in Art Therapy
Contact: Randy M. Vick, MS, ATR-BC, LCPC
Art Therapy Program
37 South Wabash Avenue
Chicago, Illinois 60603-3103
312-899-7481
arttherapy@artic.edu, <http://www.artic.edu>

Seton Hill University (initial approval 2000)
MA in Art Therapy: Specialization in Counseling; MA in Art Therapy
Contact: Nina Denninger, ATR-BC, LPC
Associate Professor and Program Director
Box 467F, Seton Hill Drive
Greensburg, Pennsylvania 15601

724-830-1047
denninger@setonhill.edu, <http://www.setonhill.edu>

Southern Illinois University at Edwardsville (initial approval 1992)
MA in Art Therapy Counseling
Contact: P. Gussie Klorer, PhD, ATR-BC, LCPC, LCSW
Director, Department of Art and Design
Box 1764, SIUE
Edwardsville, Illinois 62026-1764
618-650-3183
pklorer@siue.edu, <http://www.siue.edu/ART/areas/art_therapy/
    therapy_programs.html>

Southwestern College (initial approval 1998)
MA in Art Therapy
Contact: Kate Davis Rogers, MA, ATR, LPAT, LPCC,
Acting Program Chair, Art Therapy Program
or Tracy Meyer, Director of Admissions
PO Box 4788
Santa Fe, New Mexico 87502-4788
505-471-5756 Ext. 26 or 877-471-5756
info@swc.edu, <http://www.swc.edu>

Springfield College (initial approval 1998)
MS in Art Therapy
Contact: Leslie Abrams, PhD, LMHC, ATR-BC
Director, Graduate Art Therapy
Springfield College Visual and Performing Arts
263 Alden Street
Springfield, Massachusetts 01109-3797
413-748-3799
Leslie_R_Abrams@spfldcol.edu, <http://www.spfldcol.edu>

University of Illinois at Chicago (initial approval 1985)
MA in Art Therapy
Contact: Harriet Wadeson, PhD, ATR-BC, HLM
Art Therapy Graduate Program
M/C 36, 935 West Harrison Street
Chicago, Illinois 60607
312-996-5728
uicarttherapy@yahoo.com, <http://www.uic.edu>

University of Louisville (initial approval 1981)
MA in Art Therapy
Contact: Laura Cherry, PhD, ATR

Acting Program Director
College of Education and Human Development
Expressive Therapies Program
Louisville, Kentucky 40292
502-852-5265
etemail@louisville.edu, <http://www.louisville.edu/edu/ecpy/et/et.html>

Ursuline College (initial approval 1992)
MA in Art Therapy
Contact: Gail Rule-Hoffman, MEd, ATR-BC, CCDCIII
Art Therapy Department
2550 Lander Road
Pepper Pike, Ohio 44124
440-646-8139
grulehof@ursuline.edu, <http://www.ursuline.edu>

Wayne State University (initial approval 1994)
MEd in Art Education with Art Therapy variant; MA in Counseling with Art
    Therapy concentration, options to add Teaching Certificate in Art K-12
Contact: Holly·Feen, PhD, ATR-BC
163 Community Arts Building
Detroit, Michigan 48202
313-577-1823
hfeen@wayne.edu, <http://wayne.edu>

REFERENCES

American Art Therapy Association (2002). Definition of the Profession. Available
    at <www.art-therapy.us>.
Barker, V.I. and Brunk, B. (1991). The Role of a Creative Arts Group in the Treatment
    of Clients with Traumatic Brain Injury. *Music Therapy Perspectives, 9:* 26-31.
Buffington, A.L. and Malec, J.F. (1997). The Vocational Rehabilitation Continuum:
    Maximizing Outcomes Through Bridging the Gap from Hospital to Community-
    Based Services. *The Journal of Head Trauma Rehabilitation, 12*(5): 1-13.
Canner Hume, S. and Hitti, J. (1988). A Rationale and Model for Group Art Therapy
    with Mentally Retarded Adolescents. *A Journal of Art Therapy, 27*(1): 2-12.
DiCowden, M.A. (1987). Art Therapy: A Therapeutic Tool in Pediatric Acute and
    Rehabilitation Programs. *American Journal of Art Therapy, 26*(2): 52-56.
Fausek, D. (1997). *A Practical Guide to Art Therapy Groups.* Binghamton, NY:
    The Haworth Press.
Grace, J., Stout, J.C., and Malloy, P.F. (1999). Assessing Frontal Lobe Behavioral
    Syndromes with the Frontal Lobe Personality Scale. *Psychological Assessment
    Resources, 6*(3): 269-284.

Jacobson, E. (1938). *Progressive Relaxation.* Chicago: University of Chicago Press.

Jacobson, E. (1948). *You Must Relax: A Practical Method for Reducing the Strains of Modern Living.* New York: McGraw-Hill.

Kingsley, R.F. and Pfeuffer, D.B. (1982). Enhancing learning for the handicapped through the arts. (Report No. EC-143-133). U.S. Department of Education, National Institute of Education. (ERIC Document Reproduction Service No. ED 218 868.)

Kramer, E. (1977). *Art Therapy in a Children's Community: A Study of the Function of Art Therapy in the Treatment Program of Wiltwyck School for Boys.* New York: Schocken Books.

Landgarten, Helen B. (1981). *Clinical Art Therapy.* Bristol, PA: Brunner/Mazel.

Lazarus-Leiff, B. (1998). Art Therapy and the Aesthetic Environment As Agents for Change: A Phenomenological Investigation. Chapin Home Adult Day Health Care Center, Jamaica, New York, USA. *Art Therapy, 15*(2): 121-126.

Lezak, M.D. (1993). Newer Contributions to the Neuropsychological Assessment of Executive Functions. *The Journal of Trauma Rehabilitation, 8*(1): 24-31.

McGraw, M. (1989). Art Therapy with Brain-Injured Patients. *American Journal of Art Therapy, 28*(2): 37-44.

Miller, M.G. (1998). Art: A Creative Teaching Tool. *Academic Therapy, 22*(1): 53-56.

Murrey, G.J. and Starzinski, D. (2004). An Inpatient Neurobehavioral Rehabilitation Program for Persons with TBI: Overview of and Outcome Data for the Minnesota Neurorehabilitation Hospital. *Brain Injury, 18*(6): 519-531.

Prigatano, G. (1999). *Principles of Neuropsychological Rehabilitation.* New York: Oxford University Press.

Rosenthal, M., Christensen, B.K., and Ross, T.P. (1998). Depression Following Traumatic Brain Injury. *Archives of Physical Medicine and Rehabilitation, 79:* 90-103.

Rosner, D.I. (2000). An Exploration of the Role of Art As Therapy in Rehabilitation from Traumatic Brain Injury. The Union Inst., U.S. *Dissertation Abstracts International: Section B: The Sciences & Engineering, 60*(8-B): 3894.

Sohlberg, M.M., Mateer, C.A., and Stuss, D.T. (1993). Contemporary Approaches to the Management of Executive Control Dysfunction. *The Journal of Head Trauma Rehabilitation, 8*(1): 45-58.

Sourkes, B.M. (1991). Truth to Life: Art Therapy with Pediatric Oncology Patients and Their Siblings. *Journal of Psychosocial Oncology, 9*(2): 81-95.

Trudel, T.M., Tyron, W.W., and Purdum, C.M. (1998). Awareness of Disability and Long-Term Outcome After Traumatic Brain Injury. *Rehabilitation Psychology, 43*(4): 267-281.

Ulman, E. (1975). Therapy Is Not Enough: The Contribution of Art to General Hospital Psychiatry. In E. Ulman and P. Dachinger (Eds.), *Art Therapy in Theory and Practice* (pp. 14-32). New York: Schocken Books.

Varney, N.R. and Menefee, L. (1993). Psychosocial and Executive Deficits Following Closed Head Injury: Implications for Orbital Frontal Cortex. *The Journal of Head Trauma Rehabilitation, 8*(1): 32-44.

Very Special Arts (1993). Arts Impact Summary Report: The Effect of Arts Education on Problem Solving Skills in the Schools: A Three Year Study. Albuquerque: Very Special Arts of New Mexico.

Weaver, J. (2001). The Art of Healing. *Photo District News, 21:* 16.

Winner, Ellen (1982). *Invented Worlds: The Psychology of the Arts.* Cambridge, MA: Harvard University Press.

Wolpe, J. (1969). *The Practice of Behavior Therapy.* New York: Pergamon Press.

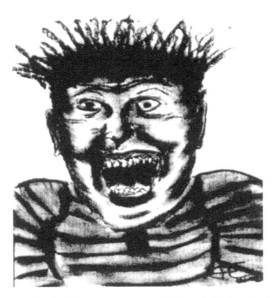

FIGURE 3.1. Artwork of a thirty-seven-year-old female TBI patient with history of self-injury, depression, and aggression. Reprinted with permission.

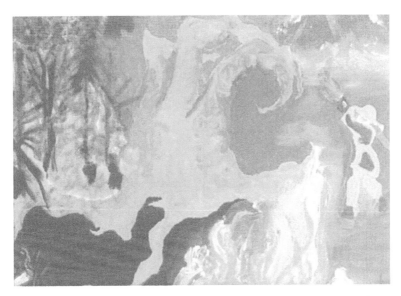

FIGURE 3.2. Artwork of a twenty-nine-year-old female TBI patient with history of assault and impulsive behaviors. Reprinted with permission.

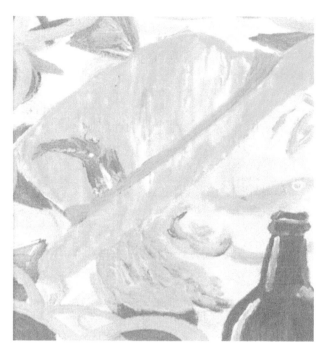

FIGURE 3.3. Artwork of a twenty-seven-year-old female TBI patient with history of chemical abuse and impulse-control disorder. Reprinted with permission.

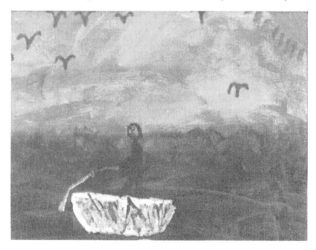

FIGURE 3.4. Artwork of a twenty-two-year-old male TBI patient with history of physical aggression and inappropriate social behaviors. Reprinted with permission.

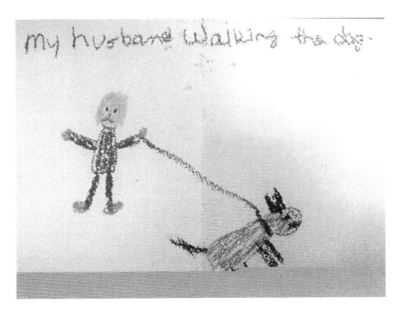

FIGURE 3.5. Artwork of a forty-two-year-old female TBI patient with sexual impulsivity issues. Reprinted with permission.

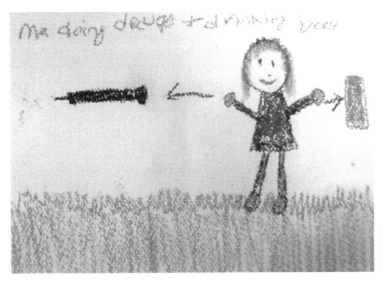

FIGURE 3.6. Second drawing from forty-two-year-old female TBI patient with sexual impulsivity issues. Reprinted with permission.

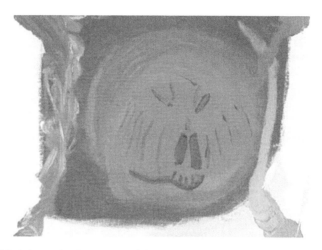

FIGURE 3.7. Artwork of a twenty-eight-year-old TBI patient who presents with a great deal of resentment and control issues regarding his relationship with his father. Reprinted with permission.

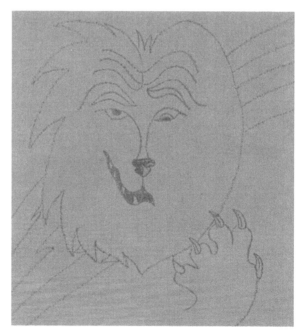

FIGURE 3.8. Artwork of a thirty-seven-year-old female TBI patient who presents with difficulty expressing feelings and coping with interpersonal relationships with family and peers. Reprinted with permission.

Chapter 4

Music Therapy for Patients with Traumatic Brain Injury

Wendy Magee
Barbara Wheeler

INTRODUCTION AND OVERVIEW

Music therapy is the use of music and musical activities in conjunction with interpersonal skills to accomplish the therapeutic goals of restoring, improving, or maintaining mental and physical health. Through carefully planned musical experiences, the client is provided with opportunities for growth. A music therapist can be described as a therapist who uses music as a tool for therapy. Music therapy has been defined by Bruscia (1998) as "a systematic process of intervention wherein the therapist helps the client to promote health, using music experiences and the relationships that develop through them as dynamic forces of change" (p. 20).

A music therapist may work with any age group and with people demonstrating a variety of physical, behavioral, or cognitive disabilities or emotional problems. As a member of a therapeutic team or as a private practitioner, the music therapist participates in the analysis of individual problems and the establishment of treatment goals before planning and carrying out music-related treatment.

Review of the Research of Music Therapy with People with Brain Injuries

The use of music therapy with people with various types of brain injuries is documented through clinical, descriptive, and research literature (AMTA, 2000a). This literature is reviewed in the following sections, and is divided into the areas in which music therapy is most frequently used: communication, cognition, physical functioning, and emotional and social functioning.

Communication

Music has long been described as a powerful tool for overcoming language disorders in people with brain damage who have limited means for verbal communication (Albert, Sparks, & Helm, 1973; Keith & Aronson, 1975; Klingler & Peter, 1963; Loebell, 1940 cited in Kennelly, Hamilton, & Cross, 2001; Rogers & Fleming, 1985). In more recent years music therapy research and clinical studies have shown that the use of music with patients with brain injuries has been found to improve verbal intelligibility (Cohen, 1992; Cohen & Masse, 1993; Kennelly et al., 2001; Pilon, McIntosh, & Thaut, 1998), rate of speech (Cohen, 1988; Cohen & Masse, 1993; Pilon et al., 1998; Kennelly et al., 2001), pitch range (Kennelly et al., 2001), speech intonation (Kennelly et al., 2001), breath capacity (Cohen & Masse, 1993; Lucia, 1987), speaking fundamental frequency variability (Cohen, 1992), coordination of respiration-phonation patterns (Lucia, 1987), and motor planning in articulatory tasks (Lucia, 1987; Magee, 1999).

Music therapy techniques can effect change for those with language disorders. They can improve expressive abilities in nonfluent aphasia (Albert et al., 1973; Baker, 2000; Kennelly et al., 2001; Lucia, 1987; Magee, 1999), facilitate word retrieval (Baker, 2000; Cohen, 1992; Cohen & Masse, 1993; Lucia, 1987; Magee, 1999), and increase meaningful and functional verbal communication even in severe aphasia (Baker, 2000).

Three groups of techniques exist that are widely used by music therapists in speech and language rehabilitation. The first of these is singing and vocal-instruction techniques. These techniques incorporate oromotor exercises set to music, breathing exercises, vocal exercises incorporating speech sounds based on hierarchy of difficulty, and song singing, all of which are systematically practiced with patients to facilitate automated responses (Basso, Capitani, & Vignolo, 1979; Cohen, 1988, 1992, 1995; Cohen & Ford, 1995; Cohen & Masse, 1993; Kennelly et al., 2001; Lucia, 1987; Magee, 1999; Rogers & Fleming, 1985).

The second group of techniques used by music therapists in speech and language rehabilitation is pacing techniques, which aim to modify speaking rate. Two different types of pacing techniques are used: *metered* rhythmic cueing, which uses a steady metronomic pulse on each syllable, and *patterned* rhythmic cueing, which uses different beat durations matched to speech prosody. Pacing techniques to improve intelligibility have had the most success in cases of severe dysarthria, but are contraindicated in cases of mild dysarthria to reduce speech rate (Pilon et al., 1998). Metered and patterned cueing are equally effective in addressing speech intelligibility (Pilon et al., 1998). There are contrasting findings comparing the effectiveness of pacing techniques and singing techniques on verbal intelligibility; however, both appear to improve speech rate (Cohen, 1988; Cohen & Masse, 1993) and speech intelligibility (Pilon et al., 1998).

The third use of music and music therapy in speech and language rehabilitation is melodic intonation therapy (MIT), which is described in more detail in Chapter 5.

Cognition

Music has been found to be effective in helping people with memory, in improving attention, and with auditory training. In addition, music therapy is used with many populations to help to deal with cognitive problems, including attention, memory, and reality orientation, and its efficacy has been documented through research (American Music Therapy Association [AMTA], 2000b). Knox and Jutai (1996) present an overview of research on the efficacy of rehabilitation for brain injury and identify ways that music-based approaches might be used in the rehabilitation of attention.

Music therapy has been used to assist in a variety of cognitive deficit areas. Gervin (1991) provided auditory cues through song lyrics with two patients with TBI (traumatic brain injury) to aid in initiating, sequencing, and motor planning in order to reduce dressing times. Lee and Baker (1997) used music therapy to improve problem solving, and Robb (1996) used music therapy to improve abstract thought.

Music therapy has been used with people who are in coma or emerging from coma. Claeys, Miller, Dalloul-Rampersad, & Kollar (1989) use improvisatory music to "increase environmental awareness, accentuate random movements, encourage vocalization, and improve reality orientation" (p. 71). Aldridge, Gustorff, & Hannich (1990) describe techniques in which improvised wordless singing is used by the therapist with coma clients, structuring the tempo, phrase length, and repetition of the music on the clients' pulses, breathing, and random movements. Boyle (Boyle & Greer, 1983; Boyle, 1995) describes the use of operant procedures with people who are in coma and reports some success. Kennelly and Edwards (1997) and Rosenfeld and Dun (1999) describe the use of music therapy with children awakening from coma.

Baker (2001) compared the effects of live, taped, and no music on agitation and orientation levels of people with TBI who were experiencing posttraumatic amnesia. She found that both live and tape-recorded music significantly reduced agitation and enhanced orientation.

The literature describing the effects of music therapy techniques on cognition in the person with brain injury provides a wealth of varying techniques for consideration. The authors recommend that clinicians working in this area give primary consideration to the patient's pathology in order to match techniques appropriately to the patient's needs and to enable the patient to achieve his or her goals.

Physical Functioning

The effectiveness of music therapy in helping to rehabilitate people who have had brain injuries has been well documented through research in the area of muscular control and movement. The majority of the studies in this area have been of neurologic music therapy (NMT), a model established in recent years specifically for working with people with neurological problems. Developed at the Center for Biomedical Research in Music at Colorado State University (http://www.colostate.edu/depts/cbrm/), this model is based on findings from empirical research that have demonstrated the effects of music on speech and language training and on cognitive training, but particularly on sensorimotor training. As a model that integrates scientific research into the biological effects of music with parallel models of nonmusic therapy treatment (Thaut, 2000), NMT has received acceptance as a proven, effective intervention for this population. It is a specialist training for people who are already trained as music therapists, and approximately 434 music therapists have been trained in NMT techniques as of June 2005.

Thaut (1999a) suggests that music therapy may be used in physical rehabilitation in two ways: movement to music and movement through music. Movement to music utilizes the organizing properties of rhythm to help individuals organize their movements. Thaut (1999a) specifies three NMT treatment methods that utilize these principles. The first is rhythmic auditory stimulation (RAS), a technique in which various forms of rhythmic beats are superimposed on movement. RAS has been used largely to improve the gait of people who have had various types of brain injuries (Hurt, Rice, McIntosh, & Thaut, 1998; McIntosh, Thaut, Rice, & Prassas, 1993, 1995; Prassas, Thaut, McIntosh, & Rice, 1997; Thaut, 1997; Thaut & McIntosh, 1992, 1999; Thaut, Hurt, & McIntosh, 1997; Thaut, McIntosh, Prassas, & Rice, 1993; Thaut, Rice, & McIntosh, 1997; Thaut, Rice, McIntosh, & Prassas, 1993; Thaut, McIntosh, Rice, & Miller, 1995; Thaut, McIntosh, & Rice, 1997). Patterned sensory enhancement (PSE) uses "rhythmic, melodic, harmonic, and dynamic aspects of music to provide temporal, spatial, and force cues for movements that reflect functional exercises and activities of daily living" (Thaut, 1999a, p. 240). PSE is applied to movements that are not rhythmic by nature and provides more than just temporal cues (Thaut, Kenyon, Hurt, McIntosh, & Hoemberg, 2002).

Utilizing movement through music, the second way that Thaut (1999a) suggests that music therapy be used in physical rehabilitation, is used in NMT through therapeutic instrumental music playing (TIMP). This technique, which has been used for many years by music therapists with people with physical problems, consists of playing musical instruments to provide structure for exercising and utilizing functional movement patterns. Elliot (1982) and Clark and Chadwick (1980) have provided guidelines for music therapists and others in adapting and using instruments to facilitate and promote functional movement patterns.

Music therapists who are not trained in NMT have also used music therapy effectively to treat physical problems of people who have had brain injuries. Cofrancesco (1985) used music therapy to improve hand-grasp strength and functional task performance with three elderly people who had experienced strokes. Staum (1983) utilized a technique in which subjects followed a sequence that involved listening to the selection, tapping a hand or other body part along with the selection, vocalizing any verbal sound to the beat, followed by walking with the music or beat, and then eliminating auditory cues. Analysis of walking yielded improvement, in some cases dramatic, for all subjects with problems of gait dysrhythmia. It also showed improvements in consistency in speed, and ratings of rhythmic, even steps, and tempo consistency and slow/fast speeds.

Cross, McLellan, Vomberg, Monga, & Monga (1984) describe their use of music in the rehabilitation of stroke patients. They observed an increase in the range and ease of movement of patients during weight-shifting activities when music with a moderate tempo was used. Tomaino (1998) also describes improving weight shifting and proprioception through music's ability to synchronize movements in a patient who had a stroke and had a gait disorder.

The effect of music techniques in the rehabilitation of physical functioning in the person with traumatic brain injury is one of the best documented in all of the music therapy literature. The research on NMT provides a solid base of evidence from which to draw when working in this field.

Emotional and Social Functioning

Music therapy is frequently acknowledged as helpful in treating the emotional and social aspects of rehabilitation from brain injuries. Much of the literature supporting the use of music therapy is descriptive, consisting primarily of case studies. Published case studies with this group describe how music therapy changes self-esteem (Purdie, 1997; Purdie & Baldwin, 1994), and self-image and identity concepts (Jochims, 1995; Magee, 1999; McMaster, 1991); decreases depression (Scheiby, 1998); increases emotional expression (Glassman, 1991; Goldberg, Hoss, & Chesna, 1988; O'Callaghan, 1993; Robb, 1996; Scheiby, 1998); improves social skills (Barker & Brunk, 1991); and improves quality of life (Scheiby, 1998). A descriptive research study by Bright and Signorelli (1999) also found an improvement in the quality of life in patients who received music therapy.

Research also supports positive emotional and social effects of music therapy with people with brain injuries. Nayak, Wheeler, Shifflet, & Agostinelli (2000) examined the efficacy of music therapy in improving mood and social interaction. They found that patients receiving music therapy were significantly more involved in their rehabilitation programs and more socially interactive, with trends suggesting that mood also improved. Magee and Davidson (2002) found that music therapy significantly improved mood states of people with a variety of neurodisabilities, including TBI and brain damage from strokes or anoxia, even after short-term intervention.

Eslinger, Stauffer, Rohrbacher, & Grattan (1993) investigated the effects of music therapy on social-emotional processing following brain injury. Results showed significant improvement in emotional empathy measures as reported by family members and friends, but not by the patients themselves. Purdie, Hamilton, & Baldwin (1997) studied the effects of twelve weeks of music therapy on long-term institutionalized patients who had had strokes, and they found that the music therapy group showed signs of being less depressed and anxious than those who did not receive music therapy. Cross et al. (1984), in a study described previously, found that posttherapy emotional measures revealed lower anxiety levels after the music therapy process began.

GOALS IN BRAIN INJURY REHABILITATION

Within brain injury rehabilitation, music therapy plays a role in working with the individual's responses as a "whole." Actively participating in music therapy allows for the assessment and rehabilitation of verbal and nonverbal communication skills, social-interaction skills, motor function, and cognitive functioning, and assists with the psychological and emotional adjustment to acquired disability. Music therapy can facilitate a more relaxed environment through the emotional and physiological effects of music. It fosters an atmosphere in which the patient can feel safe, and may offer a forum for informal and formal assessment.

Music therapists working with patients with brain damage work from many different theoretical orientations. Some focus on functional changes as the primary goals (e.g., Thaut, 1999b), whereas others work from a psychotherapeutic framework in which patients' emotional experiences are primary, often used alongside goal-oriented rehabilitation techniques (e.g., Scheiby, 1998).

Communication

Patients may be referred who have no means for verbal communication and whose ability to understand language is either impaired or not known. In such cases music therapy can provide an assessment forum that is nonfunctional and does not rely on language abilities. In this way music therapy can provide useful information for the rest of the multidisciplinary team.

For the nonverbal patient, music provides a medium for interaction and communication. Musical components form the basis for communication of basic needs and emotional states in prelinguistic human development. Preverbal infants communicate intent and immediate feeling states through pitch, melodic contour, rhythm, phrase length, dynamics, and tempo. For this reason, music is an innate medium for interaction. Despite the loss of speech or language from brain injury, musical abilities may be well preserved. Music therapy with the nonverbal patient aims to assess preverbal communication such as imitation, development, and turn-taking, and also social communication such as eye contact and other nonverbal gestures. Assessment aims to provide a baseline of the patient's communicative abilities. Goals of treatment are then set to expand upon existing abilities and to reinforce novel responses while providing a supportive environment in which the patient can experiment and explore.

Patients who have some speech may present with speech and/or language deficits. This might include language disorders such as expressive dysphasia and/or receptive dysphasia, or speech disorders such as dysarthria. Music therapy provides a forum in which the individual can work toward functional communication using a medium that is both pleasurable and rewarding, fostering an environment different from many other clinical treatment sessions. Goals of assessment are to establish the patient's level of communication abilities by monitoring his or her vocal responses, such as duration of vocal production, range of pitch, and the dynamic range the patient is able to achieve vocally. Close liaison with the speech pathologist helps in assessing the patient's general oromotor abilities and in setting realistic and achievable goals. The range of verbal sounds and words a patient is able to sing, along with the clarity of articulation of the sung sounds/words can be assessed. Goals within treatment aim to increase all aspects of vocal production, increase the range of sound/ word production, and improve the consistency and clarity of specific speech sounds within singing activities.

Cognition

Participating in music therapy involves many different aspects of cognition. Playing instruments and singing songs are complex tasks involving varied cognitive skills such as initiation, attention, concentration, short- and long-term memory, motor planning, sequencing, switching between tasks, behavioral control, motivational drive, and fluency in thinking. Merged together, deficits in these areas result in a loss of interest in the world and a reduced desire to explore oneself and the environment. This in turn leads to a loss of stimulation and impoverished creativity.

The cognitive abilities previously listed are usually impaired in the patient with brain damage and are challenged in treatment sessions of most modalities. Music, however, provides a vehicle for facilitating responses; structural components of music such as pulse, rhythm, tempo, melody, phrasing, melodic contour, harmonic direction, and dynamics compensate for cognitive deficits that inhibit the individual's ability to structure, shape, drive, and control his or her own responses. It is the music therapist's role to plan musical activities with the patient's cognitive deficits in mind, using music in ways that either compensate for the patient's cognitive difficulties or that address them. For example, problems with initiation and motivation are often overcome when beautiful and appealing musical instruments are placed within reach of the patient for exploration, or when pulse and rhythm are used to cue a response. Attention to tasks and concentration are often noted to be optimal within music therapy activities during which the patient is engaged in pleasurable and rewarding activity possessing an inherent formal structure. Familiar structures, particularly those drawing on long-term memory, such as a well-known song or repetitive pulse, are able to cue active responses and enable continuity through components such as pulse, rhythm, and melody. In this way, music therapy sessions may provide a forum for the multidisciplinary team to gauge a patient's optimal cognitive responses.

Physical Functioning

Actively participating in singing and playing requires physical activity. Playing a range of musical instruments provides opportunities for purposeful physical exploration and the development of functional movement. In particular, uni- or bilateral hand grasp, arm extension, trunk realignment, and leg extension can all be involved in making a sound on an instrument. Playing lightweight wind instruments involves the coordination of breath control and facial/oral muscles, voice production, and trunk repositioning. The goals of music therapy reflect wider multidisciplinary goals focusing on specific functional goals such as improving grasp in a particular hand through use of beaters and shaking instruments, increasing bilateral function through playing instruments, improving the coordination of movements such as walking gait, and increasing proprioceptive awareness, particularly in those patients experiencing neglect due to cognitive deficits. Music therapy may also assist with management of pain or increased muscle tone, such as for relaxation to aid in physical therapy.

Emotional Functioning

Music stimulates a range of emotional responses, manifested in feeling states and physiological responses. Patients who have acquired brain injury have considerable emotional adjustments to make, including dealing with the trauma of what has happened to them and the ensuing loss, learning to deal with changed levels of dependence and fatigue, and major changes to intimate relationships and life circumstances. The patient may present with considerable anxiety. Emotional readjustment is frequently not central to rehabilitation programs, which tend to have a functional focus. Music therapy has great potential to assist patients with adjustment to disability by providing a therapeutic outlet for emotional expression of feelings that may be too profound to explore and express verbally.

In assessment, music therapy aims to examine emotional and behavioral responses within shared musical interactions. Often, the primary goal is to improve self-esteem and feelings of well-being by increasing self-awareness and building confidence. In a safe and trusting environment, nurtured by the therapeutic relationship with the therapist, clients are encouraged to explore their abilities and challenge their limitations through creative activity. This can bring up many emotional responses, ranging from expressions of grief to expressions of joy. Goals would be for the patient to express and explore differing emotional states. A primary goal may also be to reduce anxiety and engage the patient actively in treatment. Should there be difficulties with pervasive mood states, such as low mood, the goal would be to improve mood states, particularly motivation and engagement in the wider rehabilitation program. Goals include assisting with adjustment to disability, pertinent when working with patients who have insight into their situation and are realistic about the future or who express unrealistic goals and are struggling to accept the changes in their life.

Social Functioning

Cross-culturally, music serves as a medium for social gatherings and ritualistic celebrations. It is inherently a social activity. As such, it is useful for patients with behavioral disorders stemming from brain injury to interact with others. Goals within music therapy can focus not only on the rehabilitation of social skills, but also on providing recommendations for the use of music to enhance relationships for those who show limited potential for change or development. A primary goal is therefore to assess and rehabilitate an individual's social functioning and ability to relate to the environment, and to build relationships with others. Second, music therapy offers a different experience of relating to others since active music making is a mutual experience. Singing and playing together is expressive, experienced through time and in synchronicity with another. It is a nonverbal interaction that optimizes spontaneity. For this reason, shared music making also focuses on the ability to develop and maintain relationships with others.

Patients with neurobehavioral disorders may have difficulty inhibiting behaviors that place themselves or others at risk, such as anger and aggression. Music therapy with these patients focuses on both increasing tolerance of social interaction and building tolerance to the environment by manipulating musical components to increase or decrease stimulation.

STRUCTURE WITHIN A TBI
REHABILITATION DAY TREATMENT
OR RESIDENTIAL PROGRAM

The delivery of a music therapy service can vary considerably from facility to facility depending on the resources available for a music therapist, the staff-to-patient ratio, the goals of the facility (e.g., assessment or long-term care), and the expectations of music therapy's contribution to the program. Most commonly, patients are referred to music therapy following referral criteria provided by the music therapist. Generally, goals fall under the broad categories of needs such as communication, cognition, physical functioning, and emotional or social functioning. A patient may be referred to music therapy for several reasons.

Following the referral, the music therapist undertakes an assessment of the patient to gauge a baseline of responses and estimate the potential for change or development. Assessments used in this process vary among facilities and the therapists' theoretical orientations. Many music therapy assessments are based on parallel assessments from areas such as speech, occupational, or physical therapy that focus on needs that may be addressed in music therapy (Thaut, 1999b; Thompson, Arnold, & Murray, 1990), but others formulate their own assessment instruments (Claeys et al., 1989). Duration of assessment varies among facilities, as does duration and frequency of intervention, depending on factors such as length of the patient's admission to the facility and available staff resources. Within the assessment, consideration should be given to the particular techniques that will be best suited to address the patient's needs, including whether individual or group treatment is most appropriate. The patient's overall rehabilitation program goals will be taken into consideration as part of the assessment.

At the completion of assessment, the music therapist will design a treatment plan with long-term goals broken down into short-term objectives. Priority goals as determined by the multidisciplinary team should be reflected in the music therapy treatment plan. For example, behavioral outbursts and emotional problems inhibiting a patient's engagement in therapy would indicate that facilitation of emotional expression should be foremost in the music therapist's treatment plan.

Similarly, if a patient's primary needs are to work toward functional goals such as improving upper limb movement or developing voice, then these should be reflected in the music therapy treatment plan.

Overall duration of treatment depends on such factors as the duration of the patient's admission and whether goals are achieved during the course of the therapy. When music therapy is addressing functional goals, the patient is discharged from therapy once treatment goals are achieved. In process-oriented therapy (e.g., psychotherapeutic approaches), in which music therapy is providing a forum for self-expression and emotional adjustment, the therapy may run the entire course of the patient's admission. Some facilities provide the opportunity for continuation of treatment after discharge in the form of outreach or day-service rehabilitation.

Frequency of therapy in the rehabilitation setting also varies according to whether the therapy is oriented toward functional changes or is process oriented. As in traditional psychotherapy, music therapy that aims to assist with emotional expression takes place on a weekly basis, at a regular time, and has an agreed duration, often forty-five to sixty minutes. However, therapy that is geared toward functional rehabilitation takes place more frequently, often two to five times per week. The underlying reason for increased frequency in functional rehabilitation is that the patient is literally "relearning" skills through repetition and practice. It is therefore vital that the frequency of sessions supports the patient in doing this.

Many sessions in the brain injury rehabilitation setting are held jointly with other disciplines as the patient's needs indicate. For example, when formal cognitive assessment of the patient is difficult due to the lack of appropriate standardized assessments for nonverbal patients or because the patient does not comply in other therapy sessions, a joint music therapy and psychology session may allow cognitive assessment of the patient with careful planning of activities. Similarly, when communication or physical goals are the priority, sessions are likely to be planned jointly and often run jointly with speech pathology or physical therapy, respectively. This is the case for both individual sessions in which the patient's individual goals are the focus and for group sessions in which goals are set for each individual as well as for the group as a whole. Group therapy settings can be very helpful in the rehabilitation of social functioning and to facilitate peer support and motivation to reach the goals set. Group treatment is most useful when more than one discipline is involved in planning, running, and evaluating the group. Similar to individual sessions, the frequency of group sessions varies according to the nature of the group and staff resources.

Staffing a Music Therapy Program

The music therapy program should be staffed by one or more board-certified music therapists (MT-BCs). Additional training in NMT and acceptance as an NMT Fellow are desirable for music therapists working in this area. The number of music therapy staff required will vary depending upon how the program is set up. Programs in which music therapists do extensive cotreatments with other therapists will require different staffing levels than programs in which most music therapy services are done alone. Music therapists may be assisted by, and services supplemented with, music therapy assistants. Music therapy practicum students and/or interns may also be included. Their presence not only assists in training future music therapists for this work but can also supplement the number of staff available for treatment.

Interface Among Music, Recreational, Occupational, Physical, and Speech Therapies, and Psychology Services Staff

The music therapist has a great deal to offer the multidisciplinary team in terms of providing a comprehensive therapy program that will address all aspects of the patient's psychosocial functioning. Because music is motivating, rewarding, noninvasive, and enjoyable, the patient may respond differently in a music therapy session. Findings from the music therapy session are often applicable to the broader multidisciplinary team.

The music therapist will be able to offer suggestions for using music in social and recreational activities in a way geared to meet the particular needs of the individual. Recommendations can be made for active music making or the use of music listening. The music therapist can assist with structuring groups in which music listening and the stimulation of memories to music are run by recreational therapists. Since music is such an emotionally provocative medium, it must be used sensitively, particularly with those who are dealing with the emotional consequences of such a life-changing experience as acquired brain injury. Particular recommendations can be made as to the use of musical instruments in recreational activities, including which instruments meet the patient's physical needs, how instruments should be positioned, and how the patient should be facilitated in accessing instruments.

Playing instruments in music therapy can work toward several goals. Assessment of gross and fine motor function in the hands, arms, and fingers can be undertaken by observing the patient. Cotreatment with the occupational therapist works well for this activity, during which advice on the range and nature of the patient's current motor function as well as target movement patterns can be sought. Playing instruments is a creative, motivating, and noninvasive activity to encourage upper limb movement. Joint sessions can be a place to observe the patient in a different light and plan future activities together. For the patient with profound brain damage who is undergoing sensory assessments, music therapy can be invaluable in assessing responses to auditory stimuli since it gives specific information about the optimal manipulation of different musical parameters (e.g., range of vocal pitch to use, tolerance of dynamic level) to arouse the patient and stimulate a response.

Rhythm is increasingly found to be the key in assisting with gait retraining for patients following neurological trauma or degeneration. Cotreatment with the physical therapist will help discern the patient's mobility problems and will allow the therapy to be viewed from both a motor and a musical perspective. For instance, uneven gait can be considered in terms of arrhythmia, with the music therapist playing music at a certain tempo and rhythm to assist the patient in training his or her movements and thus reduce the uneven accent and tempo of his or her gait.

The interface between speech pathology and music therapy is possibly one of the most important in the brain injury unit. As a social activity, music encourages many nonverbal communication gestures that serve as the basis for human communication and happen spontaneously in music therapy exchanges. Music and language share essential parameters, such as rhythm, pitch, contour, dynamic, duration, articulation, and tempo. Both shared and contrasting neural systems for music and language exist, and language can be rehabilitated using music. As a motivating medium, music therapy can provide a forum in which intentional communication can be assessed and rehabilitated. Speech therapy can also be supplemented with singing and voice work. The speech pathologist and the music therapist have much to offer each other. Music can facilitate and help structure responses, but the speech pathologist's experience in grading singing and language activities appropriately is essential.

Cotreatment between the psychologist and music therapist enables a better understanding of the patient's cognitive functioning and offers insight into the patient's mood state and means for emotional expression as well as the patient's inner drives and ability to relate to others in their world. Whereas the psychologist's tools are primarily words, which can be a barrier for nonverbal patients or patients with emotional/behavioral problems, the music therapist's medium provides an enabling vehicle for those who cannot participate in verbal activities or have difficulty responding to or tolerating other media. A patient's musical responses can tell us much about his or her cognitive skills, such as the ability to initiate and levels of sensory awareness, and about spontaneous responses as well as those involving executive functions. The patient's ability to inhibit and modify behavioral responses can be easily tested in music therapy activities, and therefore sessions may be useful for the psychologist to observe in order to formulate an assessment of the most challenging and "inaccessible" patients. The psychologist can also offer the music therapist interpretations of musical responses, which are relevant to understanding the patient's responses as a whole in rehabilitation. The psychologist's assistance in planning activities appropriately geared to meeting the patient's known cognitive abilities or testing unknown cognitive skills is invaluable for the music therapist working with patients with brain damage.

CASE EXAMPLES

Music therapy assessment with a nonverbal, sensory-impaired patient with behavioral problems: assessment of awareness, nonverbal communication, and supporting emotional expression.

Referral

Mrs. S. was a woman in her sixties who sustained hypoxic brain damage during a routine surgical procedure. As a consequence of brain damage, she had no active functional movement, had no means for verbal communication, was left blind, was hypersensitive to tactile stimuli, and was dependent upon others for all aspects of her care. Her only means for communication and expression were nonverbal, which were loud, distressing vocalizations that grew in intensity in volume and pitch. These vocalizations were extremely distressing for everyone around her, her family, other patients, and the staff attempting to care for her. No pattern to her vocalizing had been established, and her frequent crying prevented her from engaging in therapy. The team was unsure whether her vocal sounds were related to her environment or were due to internal pain or confusion. No reliable system of "yes" or "no" had been established. She had a diagnosis of minimally conscious state, which is a state in which the patient shows evidence of limited awareness of self or the environment, and is able to show reproducible or sustained responses to simple command following and purposeful behavior (Giacino et al., 2002).

Assessment and Intervention

Mrs. S. was referred to music therapy by speech pathology and occupational therapy at six months postinjury. The goal of the music therapy assessment was to contribute to the multidisciplinary team establishing some understanding of her crying patterns and whether these were related to stimuli in her auditory environment. She was taken by the therapist to the music therapy treatment room, which was situated off the ward for her assessment sessions. As her awareness of her surroundings could not be reliably established, sessions began with the therapist playing guitar quietly at a tempo related to her rate of breathing, and singing "hello (Mrs. S.)" repeatedly. Assessment involved listening carefully to and analyzing any vocal sounds made during the session, particularly during musical interactions, and also monitoring any behavioral changes, such as her head turning toward the sound source, her eyes closing, or any change in physical tone. Her primary way of actively participating was her vocal sounds. In particular, the musical elements of her vocalizations were noted, but also the emotional expression, such as the fluctuating dynamics, pitch, and melodic contour of her cries. The duration and articulation of her cries were also noted, differentiating between short, sharp, stabbing cries and long, legato cries. The emotional communication in her cries was noted. For example, when she was not distressed her vocalizations were calm, interactive, and related to the musical sounds offered. When distressed, the musicality of her cries changed considerably.

After the first step of listening to the patient's sounds, the therapist then reflected her sounds. That is, the musical and emotional expression of her sounds was conveyed musically and repeated back to her. At first this may have been simply mirroring the patient's sounds, but it quickly moved on to more than imitation by extending and developing her vocal sounds. The therapist attempted to match the emotional intensity of the patient's sounds. This was done through vocalizing and using the added dimension of piano harmonies. This helped to enhance and support the patient's experience. For example, if the patient's cries were distressed and expressing frustration, the therapist used discordant harmonies to provide a supportive structure for her to vocalize within. The aim of this was to empathize with her emotional expression. The primary goal in using music in this interactive way was not to calm her down but to communicate with her using her own means, saying "I can hear you and I can understand that this is what you mean and how you feel."

Within the assessment sessions, the patient responded to the therapist's mirroring of her sounds by pausing briefly in her crying to listen. Often this would then be followed by an increase in the intensity of her crying/vocalizing. Together the patient and therapist built in intensity, using a wider range of pitch, getting louder, and changing the timbral quality of both vocalized phrases. From these shared interactions during the assessment sessions, it could be established that the patient was using her vocalizing in a communicative and interactive way in these sessions. This was confirmed by her response in one session to a humorous musical gesture (a sudden bass note "plonked" at the end of a phrase). In immediate response to this, the patient laughed. Taken by surprise, the therapist offered another differing humorous musical gesture. The patient's response was similar. She did not sustain this response, but it indicated important information to the multidisciplinary team that her vocal expressive responses were related to what was going on around her. This was something that her family had been reporting but had not been observed by many members of the team in more formal assessment situations.

Assessment and Intervention Outcomes

Assessment demonstrated clearly and immediately that she moderated the musical components of her vocalizations during music therapy interactions. Following assessment, there was a short period of intervention that served as a prolonged assessment as the team continued to struggle with knowing how best to meet Mrs. S.'s needs and what her responses indicated about her levels of awareness. Music therapy sessions provided a forum for emotional expression within a supportive and boundaried space, and she usually returned to the ward quieter, more tired, and less anxious. Her family reported that she appeared less distressed after returning from music therapy. Using a musical framework for communication opportunities proved invaluable for speech pathology assessment of this client's capacity for nonverbal communication. Music therapy confirmed the family's feelings and also provided information to the team about the patient's awareness of her surroundings.

APPENDIX:
RESOURCES AND CONTACT INFORMATION

Professional Organizations and Certification

The music therapy organization in the United States is the American Music Therapy Association (AMTA) (http://www.musictherapy.org). A qualified music therapist who has completed a music therapy education and passed a professional examination can become a board-certified music therapist (MT-BC) through the Certification Board for Music Therapists (http://www.cbmt.org). Regular continuing education is required to maintain board certification. Training in neurologic music therapy is offered through the Center for Biomedical Research in Music at Colorado State University (http://www.colostate.edu/depts/cbrm/). Music therapy professional organizations exist worldwide, although training and credentialing varies from country to country. Information on music therapy and music therapy training in other countries can be obtained through the World Federation for Music Therapy (http://www.musictherapyworld.net/modules /wfmt/w_index1.htm).

Music Therapy Internship Sites/Programs

Part of the process for becoming a music therapist is to complete extensive clinical experience. The AMTA requirements specify that "every student must complete a minimum of 1200 hours of clinical training, with at least 15 percent (180 hours) in preinternship experiences and at least 75 percent (900 hours) in internship experiences. Academic institutions may opt to require more than the minimum total number of hours, and internship programs may opt to require more hours than the referring or affiliate academic institution" (AMTA, 2000b, p. 5). The preinternship clinical training is done at facilities selected by the university at which the student is studying. The internship may be done at an AMTA National Roster Internship, approved through AMTA, or at a facility approved by the university, a university-affiliated internship. Approximately 160 National Roster Internships are available in most of the states (and one in Canada) at the time of this writing.

Academic and Training Programs
in Music Therapy (Requirements)

Music therapy education in the United States is competency based. AMTA has developed a set of competencies, covering the areas of music foundations (music theory and history, composition and arranging skills, major performance medium skills, keyboard skills, guitar skills, voice skills, nonsymphonic instrumental skills, improvisation skills, conducting skills, movement skills), clinical foundations (exceptionality, principles of therapy, the therapeutic relationship), and music therapy (foundations and principles, client assessment, treatment planning, therapy implementation, therapy evaluation, documentation, termination/discharge planning, professional roles/ethics, interdisciplinary collaboration, supervision and administration, research methods). Each university can determine how to meet these competencies.

The entry level for a music therapist in the United States is a bachelor's degree, although a number of educational programs offer music therapy degrees at the master's and doctoral levels. Some music therapists earn degrees in related fields, such as counseling, special education, or speech pathology, to supplement their music therapy skills.

Web Sites and Other Media

The following music therapy Web sites have lists of publications and research. You will also find useful links to other associated Web sites on all of the following:

- American Music Therapy Association: http://www.musictherapy.org/
- The Certification Board for Music Therapists: http://www.cbmt.org
- Society for Research in Psychology of Music and Music Education: http://www.sempre.org.uk/
- Center for Biomedical Research in Music: http://www.colostate.edu /depts/cbrm/
- World Federation for Music Therapy: http://www.musictherapy world .net/modules/wfmt/w_index1.htm
- Music Therapy World: http://www.musictherapyworld.net/
- *Voices: A World Forum for Music Therapy*: http://www.voices.no/

Other music therapy resources:

- *The Arts in Psychotherapy*
- *Australian Journal of Music Therapy*
- *British Journal of Music Therapy*
- *Journal of Music Therapy*
- MMB Music and Jessica Kingsley Publishing produce many books on music therapy and provide comprehensive lists of publications
- *Music Therapy Perspectives*
- *Music Therapy Research: Quantitative and Qualitative Foundations. CD-ROM 1: 1964-1998.* American Music Therapy Association.
- *Nordic Journal of Music Therapy*

REFERENCES

Albert, M., Sparks, R., & Helm, N. (1973). Melodic Intonation Therapy for Aphasia. *Archives of Neurology, 29,* 130-131.

Aldridge, D., Gustorff, D., & Hannich, H.-J. (1990). Where Am I? Music Therapy Applied to Coma Patients. *Journal of the Royal Society of Medicine, 83,* 345-346.

American Music Therapy Association (AMTA). (2000a). *Effectiveness of Music Therapy Procedures: Documentation of Research and Clinical Practice* (3rd ed.). Silver Spring, MD: Author.

American Music Therapy Association (AMTA). (2000b). *Standards for Education and Clinical Training.* Silver Spring, MD: Author.

Baker, F. A. (2000) Modifying the Melodic Intonation Therapy Program for Adults with Severe Non-Fluent Aphasia. *Music Therapy Perspectives, 18,* 110-114.

Baker, F. A. (2001). The Effects of Live, Taped, and No Music on People Experiencing Posttraumatic Amnesia. *Journal of Music Therapy, 38,* 170-192.

Barker, V. L., & Brunk, B. (1991). The Role of a Creative Arts Group in the Treatment of Clients with Traumatic Brain Injury. *Music Therapy Perspectives, 9,* 26-31.

Basso, A., Capatini, E., & Vignolo, L. A. (1979). Influence of Rehabilitation on Language Skills in Aphasic Patients. *Archives of Neurology, 36,* 190-196.

Boyle, M. (1995). On the Vegetative State: Music and Coma Arousal Interventions. In C. A. Lee (Ed.), *Lonely Waters: Proceedings of the International Conference, Music Therapy in Palliative Care, Oxford* (pp. 163-172). Oxford: Sobell Publications.

Boyle, M. E., & Greer, R. D. (1983). Operant Procedures and the Comatose Patient. *Journal of Applied Behavioral Analysis, 16,* 3-12.

Bright, R., & Signorelli, R. (1999). Improving Quality of Life for Profoundly Brain-Impaired Clients: The Role of Music Therapy. In R. R. Pratt & D. E. Grocke (Eds.), *MusicMedicine,* Volume 3 (pp. 255-263). Parkville, Victoria, AU: Faculty of Music, The University of Melbourne.

Claeys, M. S., Miller, A. C., Dalloul-Rampersad, R., & Kollar, M. (1989). The Role of Music and Music Therapy in the Rehabilitation of Traumatically Brain Injured Clients. *Music Therapy Perspectives, 6,* 71-77.

Clark, C., & Chadwick, D. (1980). *Clinically Adapted Instruments for the Multiply Handicapped.* St. Louis, MO: MMB Music.

Cofrancesco, E. M. (1985). The Effect of Music Therapy on Hand Grasp Strength and Functional Task Performance in Stroke Patients. *Journal of Music Therapy, 23,* 129-145.

Cohen, N. S. (1988). The Use of Superimposed Rhythm to Decrease the Rate of Speech in a Brain-Damaged Adolescent. *Journal of Music Therapy, 25,* 85-93.

Cohen, N. S. (1992). The Effect of Singing Instruction on the Speech Production of Neurologically Impaired Persons. *Journal of Music Therapy, 29,* 87-102.

Cohen, N. S. (1995). The Effect of Vocal Instruction and Visi-Pitch Feedback on the Speech of Persons with Neurogenic Communication Disorders: Two Case Studies. *Music Therapy Perspectives, 13,* 70-75.

Cohen, N. S., & Ford, J. (1995) The Effect of Musical Cues on the Nonpurposive Speech of Persons with Aphasia. *Journal of Music Therapy, 32,* 46-57.

Cohen, N. S., & Masse, R. (1993). The Application of Singing and Rhythmic Instruction As a Therapeutic Intervention for Persons with Neurogenic Communication Disorders. *Journal of Music Therapy, 30,* 81-99.

Cross, P., McLellan, M., Vomberg, E., Monga, M., & Monga, T. N. (1984). Observations on the Use of Music in Rehabilitation of Stroke Patients. *Physiotherapy Canada, 36,* 197-201.

Elliott, B. (1982). *Guide to the Selection of Musical Instruments with Respect to Physical Ability and Disability.* St. Louis, MO: MMB Music.

Eslinger, P., Stauffer, J. W., Rohrbacher, M., & Grattan, L. M. (1993). Music Therapy and Brain Injury. Report to the Office of Alternative Medicine at the NIH. Grant Number: R21RR09415.

Gervin, A. P. (1991). Music Therapy Compensatory Technique Utilizing Song Lyrics During Dressing to Promote Independence in the Patient with a Brain Injury. *Music Therapy Perspectives, 9,* 87-90.

Giacino, J. T., Ahswal, S., Childs, N., Cranford, R., Jennett, B., Katz, D. I., Kelly, J. P., Rosenberg, J. H., Whyte, J., Zafonte, R. D., & Zasler, N. D. (2002). The Minimally Conscious State: Definition and Diagnostic Criteria. *Neurology, 58,* 349-353.

Glassman, L. R. (1991). Music Therapy and Bibliotherapy in the Rehabilitation of Traumatic Brain Injury: A Case Study. *The Arts in Psychotherapy, 18,* 149-156.

Goldberg, F. S., Hoss T. M., & Chesna, T. (1988). Music and Imagery As Psychotherapy with a Brain Damaged Patient: A Case Study. *Music Therapy Perspectives, 5,* 41-45.

Hurt, C. P., Rice, R. R., McIntosh, G. C., & Thaut, M. H. (1998). Rhythmic Auditory Stimulation in Gait Training for Patients with Traumatic Brain Injury. *Journal of Music Therapy, 35,* 228-241.

Jochims, S. (1995). Emotional Processes of Coping with Disease in the Early Stages of Acquired Cerebral Lesions. *The Arts in Psychotherapy, 22,* 21-30.

Keith, R. L., & Aronson, A. E. (1975). Singing As Therapy for Apraxia of Speech and Aphasia: Report of a Case. *Brain and Language, 2,* 483-488.

Kennelly, J., & Edwards, J. (1997). Providing Music Therapy to the Unconscious Child in the Paediatric Intensive Care Unit. *Australian Journal of Music Therapy, 8,* 18-29.

Kennelly, J., Hamilton, L., & Cross, J. (2001). The Interface of Music Therapy and Speech Pathology in the Rehabilitation of Children with Acquired Brain Injury. *Australian Journal of Music Therapy, 12,* 13-20.

Klingler, H., & Peter, D. (1963). Techniques in Group Singing for Aphasics. *Music Therapy 1962, 12,* 109-112.

Knox, R., & Jutai, J. (1996). Music-Based Rehabilitation of Attention Following Brain Injury. *Canadian Journal of Rehabilitation, 9,* 169-181.

Lee, K., & Baker, F. (1997). Toward Integrating a Holistic Rehabilitation System: The Implications for Music Therapy. *Australian Journal of Music Therapy, 8,* 30-37.

Lucia, C. M. (1987). Toward Developing a Model of Music Therapy Intervention in the Rehabilitation of Head Trauma Patients. *Music Therapy Perspectives, 4,* 34-39.

Magee, W. (1999). Music Therapy Within Brain Injury Rehabilitation: To What Extent Is Our Clinical Practice Influence by the Search for Outcomes? *Music Therapy Perspectives, 17,* 20-26.

Magee, W. L., & Davidson, J. W. (2002). The Effect of Music Therapy on Mood States in Neurological Patients: A Pilot Study. *Journal of Music Therapy, 39,* 20-29.

McIntosh, G. C., Thaut, M. H., Rice, R. R., & Prassas, S. G. (1993). Auditory Rhythmic Cuing in Gait Rehabilitation with Stroke Patients. *Canadian Journal of Neurological Sciences, 20,* 168.

McIntosh, G. C., Thaut, M. H., Rice, R. R., & Prassas, S. G. (1995). Rhythmic Facilitation of Gait Kinematics in Stroke Patients. *Journal of Neurologic Rehabilitation, 9,* 131.

McMaster, N. (1991). Reclaiming a Positive Identity: Music Therapy in the Aftermath of a Stroke. In K. E. Bruscia (Ed.), *Case Studies in Music Therapy* (pp. 547-560). Gilsum, NH: Barcelona Publishers.

Nayak, S., Wheeler, B. L., Shiflett, S. C., & Agostinelli, S. (2000). The Effect of Music Therapy on Mood and Social Interaction Among Individuals with Acute Traumatic Brain Injury and Stroke. *Rehabilitation Psychology, 45,* 274-283.

O'Callaghan, C. C. (1993). Communicating with Brain-Impaired Palliative Care Patients Through Music Therapy. *Journal of Palliative Care, 9*(4), 53-55.

Pilon, M. A., McIntosh, K. W., & Thaut, M. H. (1998). Auditory vs. Visual Speech Timing Cues as External Rate Control to Enhance Verbal Intelligibility in Mixed Spastic-Ataxic Dysarthric Speakers: A Pilot Study. *Brain Injury, 12,* 793-803.

Prassas, S., Thaut, M. H., McIntosh, G. C., & Rice, R. (1997). Effect of Auditory Rhythmic Cueing on Gait Kinematic Parameters of Stroke Patients. *Gait & Posture, 6,* 218-223.

Purdie, H. (1997). Music Therapy in Neurorehabilitation: Recent Developments and New Challenges. *Critical Reviews in Physical and Rehabilitation Medicine, 9*(3&4), 205-217.

Purdie, H., & Baldwin, S. (1994). Music Therapy: Challenging Low Self-Esteem in People with a Stroke. *British Journal of Music Therapy, 8*(2), 19-24.

Purdie, H., Hamilton, S., & Baldwin, S. (1997). Music Therapy: Facilitating Behavioral and Psychological Change in People with Stroke—A Pilot Study. *International Journal of Rehabilitation Research, 20,* 325-327.

Robb, S. L. (1996). Techniques in Song Writing: Restoring Emotional and Physical Well Being in Adolescents Who Have Been Traumatically Injured. *Music Therapy Perspectives, 14,* 30-37.

Rogers, G. P., & Fleming, P. (1985). Rhythm and Music in Speech Therapy for the Neurologically Impaired. *Music Therapy, 1,* 33-38.

Rosenfeld, J. V., & Dun, B. (1999). Music Therapy in Children with Severe Traumatic Brain Injury. In R. R. Pratt & D. E. Grocke (Eds.), *MusicMedicine,* Volume 3 (pp. 35-46). Melbourne, AU: The University of Melbourne

Scheiby, B. B. (1998). Music As Symbolic Expression: Analytic Music Therapy. In D. J. Wiener (Ed.), *Beyond Talk Therapy* (pp. 263-285). Washington, DC: American Psychological Association.

Sparks, R., Helm, N., & Albert, M. (1974). Aphasia Rehabilitation Resulting from Melodic Intonation Therapy. *Cortex, 10,* 303-316.

Sparks, R. W., & Holland, A. L. (1976). Method: Melodic Intonation Therapy for Aphasia. *Journal of Speech and Hearing Disorders, 41,* 287-297.

Staum, M. J. (1983). Music and Rhythmic Stimuli in the Rehabilitation of Gait Disorders. *Journal of Music Therapy, 20,* 69-87.

Thaut, M. H. (1997). Rhythmic Auditory Stimulation in Rehabilitation of Movement Disorders: A Review of Current Research. In D. J. Schneck & J. K. Schneck (Eds.), *Music in Human Adaptation* (pp. 223-230). Blacksburg: Virginia Polytechnic Institute and State University.

Thaut, M. H. (1999a). Music Therapy in Neurological Rehabilitation. In W. B. Davis, K. E. Gfeller, & M. H. Thaut (Eds.), *An Introduction to Music Therapy: Theory and Practice* (2nd ed.) (pp. 221-247). Boston: McGraw-Hill.

Thaut, M. H. (1999b). *Training Manual for Neurologic Music Therapy.* Ft. Collins, CO: Center for Biomedical Research in Music.

Thaut, M. H. (2000). *A Scientific Model of Music in Therapy and Medicine.* San Antonio, TX: IMR Press.

Thaut, M. H., Hurt, C. P., & McIntosh, G. C. (1997). Rhythmic Entrainment of Gait Patterns in Traumatic Brain Injury Rehabilitation. *Journal of Neurologic Rehabilitation, 11,* 131.

Thaut, M. H., Kenyon, G. P., Hurt, C. P., McIntosh, G. C., & Hoemberg, V. (2002). Kinematic Optimization of Spatiotemporal Patterns in Paretic Arm Training with Stroke Patients. *Neuropsychologia, 40,* 1073-1081.

Thaut, M. H., & McIntosh, G. C. (1992). Effect of Auditory Rhythm on Temporal Stride Parameters and EMG Patterns in Normal and Hemiparetic Gait. *Neurology, 42,* 208.

Thaut, M. H., & McIntosh, G. C. (1999). Music Therapy and Mobility Training with the Elderly: A Review of Current Research. *Care Management Journals, 1,* 71-74.

Thaut, M. H., McIntosh, G. C., Prassas, S. G., & Rice, R. R. (1993). Effect of Rhythmic Cuing on Temporal Stride Parameters and EMG Patterns in Hemiparetic Gait of Stroke Patients. *Journal of Neurological Rehabilitation, 7,* 9-16.

Thaut, M. H., McIntosh, G. C., & Rice, R. R. (1997). Rhythmic Facilitation of Gait Training in Hemiparetic Stroke Rehabilitation. *Journal of Neurological Sciences, 151,* 207-212.

Thaut, M. H., McIntosh, G. C., Rice, R. R., & Miller, R. A. (1995). Rhythmic Auditory-Motor Training in Gait Rehabilitation with Stroke Patients. *Journal of Stroke and Cerebrovascular Disease, 5,* 100-101.

Thaut, M. H., Rice, R. R., & McIntosh, G. C. (1997). Rhythmic Facilitation of Gait Training in Hemiparetic Stroke Rehabilitation. *Journal of Neurological Sciences, 151,* 7-12.

Thaut, M. H., Rice, R. R., McIntosh, G. C., & Prassas, S. G. (1993). The Effect of Auditory Rhythmic Cuing on Stride and EMG Patterns in Hemiparetic Gait of Stroke Patients. *Physical Therapy, 73,* 107.

Thompson, A. B., Arnold, J. C., & Murray, S. E. (1990). Music Therapy Assessment of the Cerebrovascular Accident Patient. *Music Therapy Perspectives, 8,* 23-29.

Tomaino, C. M. (1998). Music and Memory: Accessing Residual Function. In C. M. Tomaino (Ed.), *Clinical Applications of Music in Neurologic Rehabilitation* (pp. 19-27). St. Louis, MO: MMB Music.

Chapter 5

Melodic Intonation Therapy with Brain-Injured Patients

Susan Schaefer
Martha A. Murrey
Wendy Magee
Barbara Wheeler

INTRODUCTION AND OVERVIEW

Sparks and colleagues (Sparks et al., 1974; Sparks and Holland, 1976) theorized that combining basic language with musical forms would facilitate cooperation in the brain between the right and left hemisphere. They called this *melodic intonation therapy* (MIT). In the studies it was determined that although the final integration of language function occurs in the dominant left hemisphere, the right hemisphere also possesses an auditory vocabulary. In addition, the right hemisphere was found to be the area in which the supra-segmental aspects of language (stress and intonational contours) are processed. Since the right hemisphere is also dominant for music, Sparks and colleagues (1974) theorized that this cooperation between the two hemispheres would tap the latent language abilities of the right hemisphere. MIT is typically utilized with aphasic persons with significant speech deficits. The preserved skills of singing and of recitation of familiar statements/phrases and profanity initially started the research in this area.

Basically, MIT is a structured language rehabilitative program for people with expressive aphasia, a language disorder. It is typically employed by speech pathologists or music therapists. MIT utilizes a person's ability to produce sung-type verbalizations even when he or she is not able to speak, and employs a structured program in which intoned sentences that have the same rhythm and inflection as speech are repeatedly presented to the patient. Once the patient's responses are consistent, the melody is gradually faded away. The approach was initially developed and investigated by speech pathologists and other nonmusic therapists (Albert et al., 1973, 1974; Sparks et al., 1974; Sparks and Holland, 1976), but it is also described in the music therapy literature (Kennelly et al., 2001; Lucia, 1987; Magee, 1999; Thaut, 1999a,b). Modified forms of MIT have also been found to be successful with people with severe aphasia who did not respond to conventional MIT (Baker, 2000). This involves modifying the musical structure so that phrases have greater melodic structure and a wider pitch range, with the client being required to produce only a target word rather than an entire phrase.

GENERAL PRINCIPLES OF MIT
IN REHABILITATING FUNCTIONAL SPEECH
AND EMOTIONAL EXPRESSION

With MIT, several principles of language therapy are adhered to. The first principle involves gradual progression of length and difficulty of tasks. As the tasks progress in length, participation of the clinician decreases. In addition, latency between the presentation and the response is widened. The second principle involves the use of functional high-probability utterances. The material should also be familiar since this could trigger a recall of premorbid language skills. The third principle involves focusing on the content of the response and its semantic content. As the length of stimulus increases, exact word-for-word repetitions may no longer be necessary.

A structured presentation is used in MIT. As noted previously, this is based on three elements of the spoken language: the tempo and rhythm of the utterance, melodic line or variation of pitch, and the points of stress for emphasis. First, the tempo is lengthened to a more lyrical utterance. Second, the varying pitch of the speech is reduced and patterned into a melody involving the constant pitch of the intoned notes. Third, the rhythm and stress are exaggerated for purposes of emphasis. This can involve increased loudness and elevation of words. The last step is a return to normal speech prosody. Longer delays are imposed by the therapist, before the patient is permitted to respond. In addition, more spontaneous and appropriate verbal speech is anticipated.

The original hierarchy of MIT is highly structured, with gradual progression of difficulty. Much discussion has occurred regarding whether it is necessary to follow this highly structured approach or if less structured intervention strategies could work. The following is a quick-reference hierarchy guide for MIT applications as outlined by Sparks and Deck (1986).

Level I

Single Step

Clinician hums melody twice with hand tapping each beat/syllable.
Clinician and patient hum and tap melody twice, in unison.
Clinician fades humming as tapping continues.

Scoring and progression:

Acceptable: proceed to next melody.
Unacceptable: repeat.

Level II

Step 1

Clinician hums melody and intones sentence, with hand tapping.
Clinician signals the patient.
Clinician and patient intone sentence in unison, with hand tapping.

Scoring and progression:

Acceptable: 1 point; proceed to step 2.
Unacceptable: discontinue; return to step 1.

Step 2

> Clinician hums melody and intones same sentence, with hand tapping.
> Clinician signals patient.
> Clinician and patient intone the sentence in unison, with hand tapping.
> Clinician fades.

Scoring and progression:

> Acceptable: 1 point; proceed to step 3.
> Unacceptable: discontinue progression for sentence.

Step 3

> Clinician intones same sentence, with hand tapping.
> Clinician signals patient.
> Clinician and patient intone the sentence in unison, with hand tapping.
> Patient intones sentence.
> Clinician intones cue, if necessary.

Scoring and progression:

> Acceptable without cue: 2 points; proceed to step 4 with same sentence.
> Acceptable with cue: 1 point; proceed to step 4 with same sentence.
> Unacceptable: discontinue progression with sentence.

Step 4

> Clinician intones "What did you say?"
> Clinician signals patient.
> Patient repeats the intoned sentence.
> Clinician intones cue, if necessary.

Scoring and progression:

> Acceptable without cue: 2 points.

Acceptable with cue: 1 point.
Proceed to level III, step 1.

Level III

Step 1

Clinician intones sentence, with hand tapping.
Clinician and patient intone the sentence in unison, with hand
  tapping.
Clinician fades.

Scoring and progression:

Acceptable: 1 point; proceed to step 2 with same sentence.
Unacceptable: discontinue progression for sentence.

Step 2

Clinician intones same sentence.
Clinician signals patient to wait.
Clinician signals patient to continue after one to two seconds.
Patient repeats the sentence, with hand tapping.
Return to step 1 if the patient fails. Retrial step 2.

Scoring and progression:

Acceptable without returning to step 1: 2 points; proceed to step
  3 with same sentence.
Acceptable after repetition of step 1: 1 point; proceed to step 3
  with same sentence.
Unacceptable after repetition of step 1: discontinue progression
  for sentence.

Step 3

Clinician intones a question.
Clinician signals patient.
Patient gives an appropriate answer, intoned or spoken.
Return to step 2 if the patient fails. Retrial of step 3.

Scoring and progression:

Acceptable without returning to step 2: 2 points.
Acceptable after repetition of step 2: 1 point.
Proceed to level IV, step 1.

Level IV

Please note: During this level, speech is modified to halfway between speech and singing. This is known as *sprechgesang*, as identified by Sparks and Holland, 1976, and refers to the fading of the melodic intonation. The exaggerated tempo, rhythm, and points of stress in sprechgesang are the same as in the original sentences, but there is more variation in pitch. The utterance is lyrical, but spoken rather than sung.

Step 1

Clinician intones sentence, with hand tapping.
Clinician signals patient to wait.
Clinician presents the sentence twice, with a mix of lyrical quality and spoken word along with hand tapping.
Clinician and patient intone sentence, in unison.
Return to the clinician presentation if the patient cannot make the transfer to closer speech.
Retrial of clinician and patient in unison, with hand tapping.

Scoring and progression:

Acceptable: 2 points; proceed to step 2 with same sentence.
Acceptable after returning to clinician presentation: 1 point; proceed to step 2 with same sentence.
Unacceptable: discontinue progression for sentence.

Step 2

Clinician presents the same sentence in a mixture of speech and melody, with hand tapping.
Clinician signals patient to wait.
After two to three seconds, patient repeats the sentence, with hand tapping.

Return to step 1 if patient fails, with retrial of step 2.

Scoring and progression:

Acceptable without returning to step 1: 2 points; proceed to step 3.
Unacceptable: discontinue progression for sentence.

Step 3

No hand tapping.
Clinician presents same sentence twice in normal speech prosody.
Clinician signals patient to wait two to three seconds.
Clinician signals patient to repeat the sentence.
Patient repeats the sentence in normal speech prosody.
Return to the beginning of step 3 if the patient fails.
Retrial of patient repeating.

Scoring and progression:

Acceptable without returning to step 2: 2 points; proceed to step 4 with the same sentence.
Acceptable after returning to step 2: 1 point; proceed to step 4 with same sentence.
Unacceptable: discontinue progression of sentence.

Step 4

Clinician questions patient about sentences produced, stimulating spontaneous, accurate responses targeted in therapy.
Patient answers appropriately.
Return to Step 3 if response is unacceptable.
Clinician asks questions about associated information.
Patient answers appropriately.

Scoring and progression:

Answers without returning to step 3: 2 points.
Responds appropriately to associated information questions: 3 bonus points.

Proceed to next sentence.

Level V

Gradual progression of phasing out MIT. Normal speech prosody is repeated, with a focus on use of melodic intonation independently, especially in difficult speaking situations.

CASE EXAMPLES

In the following cases, the specific levels were not always strictly followed, but rather portions of the principles were used to specifically address and facilitate the skills demonstrated by each patient. In the four cases discussed, it will be shown that MIT has been beneficial for some traumatically brain-injured patients.

Case Example 1

Mr. A., a thirty-one-year-old male with a young family, was admitted to the hospital seven months after an injury sustained in a traffic accident. He presented with considerable damage to the left hemisphere of his brain, resulting in expressive and receptive aphasia. He was aphonic and unable to voice upon admission. He was hemiplegic on his right side, although he had purposeful movement in his left arm. All verbal communication by Mr. A. was accompanied by gestures and pointing, and his only means of expressive communication was facial movements. He had previously been a keen amateur musician, playing guitar and piano and singing solo parts in musicals with an amateur theater group.

One year postinjury, Mr. A. attended two different joint disciplinary groups that addressed nonverbal communication and social skills using simple turn-taking activities before commencing individual therapy one year postinjury. He was referred for individual therapy at this time because he was poorly motivated to participate in his wider therapy and was starting to show behavioral problems that the team felt were due to increasing insight and resulting low mood. The long-term aim was to maximize the use of his musical abilities to facilitate nonverbal expression through musical improvisation.

Assessment

In the assessment it emerged that Mr. A. would not engage with playing instruments. The goal of emotional expression through instrumental improvisation was abandoned since he shook his head and frowned when shown the instruments. In an effort to engage him, familiar songs were played and it was noted that he mouthed the words to the songs but could not make any vocal sound. He was able to comprehend written material at a one-word level, and so was asked to select a mood from a short written list that best identified how he was feeling at the start and end of each session. This was to establish whether music therapy was facilitating a change of mood. The aims at this stage were to motivate and increase his participation in rehabilitation, provide opportunities for exploration of mood, and provide alternative means of expression. Although MIT is a technique that is most successful with patients with expressive aphasia rather than receptive aphasia, his responses to familiar songs suggested that song-based techniques might be useful. Close liaison with speech pathology was ensured to plan appropriate and achievable treatment goals.

In the second week of his assessment, he sang the last word in each phrase of a familiar song and sang the therapist's name within a structured welcome song. Although his articulation was poor and his voice was weak, he was able to approximate the pitch and range of verbal sounds in his sung words. The melodic, rhythmic, structural, and verbal elements constituting the framework of the song were providing the cue he needed to prompt verbalization. Although he was able to produce words when singing, he remained unable to do so without the musical framework.

Intervention

A therapy program was then planned with the main foci being communication and emotional expression. In close collaboration with the speech pathologist, the short-term communication goal became to maximize his vocalization to familiar songs. This was broken down into two steps. The first was to encourage him initially to sing the final words of phrases relying on musical prompts only. The second was to encourage him to sing as many words of each phrase as he could. He also chose different family members' names to sing in the initial hello song. Singing exercises on specific speech sounds and sound combinations were introduced to improve his articulation and oromotor skills. The speech pathologist identified which speech sounds were most achievable, and the music therapist composed creative singing exercises with which to practice sounds. Breathing and singing exercises monitored his developing breath control, and he was often noted to spontaneously improve his trunk positioning and posture in his wheelchair when singing. Furthermore, it became apparent that active participation in singing tasks elevated his mood. The success he experienced, combined with developing insight, led to emotional responses such as pleasure, but also frustration when his attempts were unsuccessful.

Despite his remarkable results when singing, the complexity of his communication impairments caused him to remain largely nonverbal without music due to dyspraxia, word-finding deficits, and perseveration problems. The activity of singing well-consolidated songs provided an automated motor sequence that overcame each of these difficulties. He remained unable to produce any spoken output at this stage.

At this point, fifteen months postinjury, a program of modified MIT with joint music and speech and language therapy commenced. As described earlier, this is a technique in which short functional phrases are repeatedly sung to a melody that imitates speech prosody. The overall goal was to increase the number of words he was able to use. The phrases learned by Mr. A. were between three and five words long, of a functional nature, and used in other settings within his program. In this way, the practical use of MIT and its carryover could be observed. However, because of word-finding and initiation difficulties, Mr. A. remained largely dependent on the context and on others in his attempts to communicate. Through simple, nonstandardized musical tests, it was assessed that his rhythmic skills remained more intact than his other musical skills. This knowledge was transferred to his communication program, and it was found that by tapping a slow pulse on his leg he was able to cue himself to produce practiced phrases more easily and independently than without tapping. Both metered and rhythmic cueing were assessed, with successful results to each of the techniques. Both types of pacing techniques were used to aid his initiation of verbal production.

Outcomes of Therapy

Mr. A. used all of the techniques previously described to access the practiced phrases outside of the music therapy session. Each time that he was successful in communicating something, he was thrilled and surprised. He attended individual music therapy for three months, including MIT during the last month. At the time of discharge, seventeen months postinjury, he was inconsistently able to produce a few short functional verbal phrases that had been practiced using MIT, and he was continuing to show considerable change and improvement in his general functional abilities. He used songs as a way of expressing a range of emotional states, and within sessions indicated most often that he felt "sad" and "fed up." It seemed that his use of songs offered him a chance to explore particular emotions and played a crucial role in motivating him through an emotionally difficult period by providing him with an expressive outlet. Joint music therapy and speech pathology sessions therefore were a place to experience success, but also a place to express sadness and a range of emotional responses.

Case Example 2

This case involved a thirty-six-year-old woman who had been involved in a head-on automobile accident. She was employed as a librarian and lived with her significant other and her sixteen-year-old daughter. At the time she was admitted to the rehab hospital, she had already underwent six months of rehabilitation at another site. She offered no spontaneous speech and presented with severe attentional deficits. She was initially able to maintain sustained attention for a maximum of only two minutes per session, and was unable to consistently follow visual stimuli across midline. Auditory comprehension was limited with minimal responses, despite maximum cueing. Mobility was limited and required two-person assistance with all tasks and total assistance with all daily grooming/feeding tasks. During the course of therapy, aspects of MIT were utilized. Attentional training was provided. The interdisciplinary team, including physical, occupational, and speech therapy, utilized MIT during the course of treatment. For example, as physical therapy tasks were completed, the repetition was often sung in a rhythm. The patient demonstrated good progress with this intervention. Unison repetition was initiated with the patient demonstrating attempts to vocalize. She began to imitate the simple sentences and showed improved attentional skills to task and offered occasional vocal response to questions. Hand tapping also facilitated imitation. Upon discharge, she was able to offer one- to two-word answers to moderate-demand questions, and to state basic needs 75 percent of the time. Though she did not return to her prior independent level of functioning, MIT provided her a means to communicate basic needs to her caregivers. She was able to return home and live with her mother.

Case Example 3

The patient in this case was admitted to the rehab facility four months post-TBI (traumatic brain injury). She was involved in a car accident that caused a head injury from hitting the windshield and a metal steering-wheel lock (which was projected from the back seat into the back of her skull). Upon admittance, she had a Rancho Los Amigos scale score of level one (no response). She would respond minimally to stimuli with general eye opening and occasional verbalization of a moan. Music was introduced at specific times during the day (9:00 to 9:30 a.m.), with therapy scheduled at other times. During therapeutic sessions, simple commands were introduced with a specific rhythm/pattern. This was continued for one to two months. She began to turn her head to the rhythmic pattern, and began to attempt some purposeful response motorically with range of motion tasks. She also began to attempt verbal responses to stimuli, though this was often unintelligible. As therapy progressed she was able to answer simple questions with yes or no responses when asked in a rhythmic tone. Her family was also able to utilize this method to communicate basic needs with her.

Case Example 4

This case demonstrates the use of melodic intonation therapy with a patient that suffered a TBI, and then a cerebrovascular accident. He was found in his house approximately six hours after the traumas. He was a fifty-seven-year-old male who lived alone and worked as a welder in a rural community. Upon admittance, he did not offer any vocalizations. Auditory comprehension and receptive language skills were judged to be minimally to moderately impaired, and expressive language skills were severely impaired.

During the course of treatment the patient improved with MIT. The traditional series was initiated with simple intonation of phrases and sentences. These were progressively increased in length and complexity with stress points added. Humming and hand tapping was also patterned. After one week he began to be able to hum independently with cues or examples. Unison patterning was initiated, with the patient demonstrating increased ability as therapy progressed. The therapists began to fade their participation in the rote and rhythmic sentences. Hand tapping was continued during this stage. As he improved with the rote/routine sentences, additional sentences were added. Sound substitutions were noted approximately 25 to 50 percent of the time. At this time he still could not spontaneously respond to personal or general questions from his family or staff, although increased verbal responses were noted. These responses were unintelligible at first and often perseverative. Sentence-completion/fill-in-the-blank statements were initiated, with hand tapping and rhythmic presentation with good response noted. As the patient progressed with accuracy, the hand tapping was reduced. Increased usage of this technique was encouraged by therapists, nurses, and his family. As this occurred, he was able to demonstrate increased response to stimuli that required one to four words to complete statements. Staff would begin by asking him open-ended questions with simple leader phrases noting good responses. For example, the staff would ask, "Do you want to have a drink?" which would be followed with a leader phrase such as, "I would like . . ." Upon conclusion of therapy, the patient was able to state basic needs by completing these simple leader phrases. He was able to offer spontaneous phrases utilizing rhythm independently fourteen to twenty-five times a day per staff and family interactions.

Melodic intonation therapy has many different levels and techniques. Modifications can and should be made to meet the individual patient's needs when using MIT with the TBI patient. However, functional communication for the significantly impaired is paramount in the overall plan for each patient.

REFERENCES

Albert, M., Sparks, R., & Helm, N. (1973). Melodic Intonation Therapy for Aphasia. *Archives of Neurology, 29,* 130-131.

Baker, F.A. (2000). Modifying the Melodic Intonation Therapy Program for Adults with Severe Non-Fluent Aphasia. *Music Therapy Perspectives, 18,* 100-114.

Kennelly, J., Hamilton, L., & Cross, J. (2001). The Interface of Music Therapy and Speech Pathology in the Rehabilitation of Children with Acquired Brain Injury. *Australian Journal of Music Therapy, 12,* 13-20.

Lucia, C.M. (1987). Toward Developing a Model of Music Therapy Intervention in the Rehabilitation of Head Trauma Patients. *Music Therapy Perspectives, 4,* 34-39.

Magee, W. (1999). Music Therapy Within Brain Injury Rehabilitation: To What Extent Is Our Clinical Practice Influenced by the Search for Outcomes? *Music Therapy Perspectives, 17,* 20-26.

Sparks, R. and Deck, J. (1986). Melodic Intonation Therapy. In R. Chapey (Ed.), *Language Intervention Strategies in Adult Aphasia* (pp. 320-332). Baltimore: Williams & Wilkins.

Sparks, R., Helm, N., and Albert, M. (1974). Aphasia Rehabilitation Resulting from Melodic Intonation Therapy. *Cortex, 10,* 303-313.

Sparks, R.W. and Holland, A.L. (1976). Method: Melodic Intonation Therapy for Aphasia. *Journal of Speech and Hearing Disorders, 41,* 287-297.

Thaut, M.H. (1999a). Music Therapy in Neurological Rehabilitation. In W.B. Davis, K.E. Gfeller, & M.H. Thaut (Eds.), *An Introduction to Music Therapy: Theory and Practice* (pp. 221-247). Boston: McGraw-Hill.

Thaut, M.H. (1999b). *Training Manual for Neurologic Music Therapy.* Ft. Collins, CO: Center for Biomedical Research in Music.

Chapter 6

Recreational Therapy Program for Patients with Traumatic Brain Injury

Mark Sell
Gregory J. Murrey

INTRODUCTION AND OVERVIEW

Much has been written about the importance of recreational leisure in a person's daily existence. People in today's society are given more leisure time than ever before. How this time is used in therapy with various disability groups has been the focus of relatively modern treatment modalities and has been recognized as an integral part of modern holistic therapies. The evolution of therapeutic recreation is a direct result of the value placed on it within various medical rehabilitation programs for different disability groups. Since leisure is often viewed as play without tangible work and is often equated with unproductive activity, its worth has often been dismissed in the therapeutic setting. However, research on the benefits of recreational therapy have dispelled this concept of low value.

Recreational therapy has the same foundation as any traditional therapy program and has benefits in every facet of human recovery from trauma or illness. Depending on which areas of the brain are damaged, brain injury can produce losses in movement, sensation, communication, intellect, and memory (Bullock & Mahon, 2001). The physical benefits are self-evident in practically any recreational activity in which a person participates and can include reduction of numerous health problems such as high blood pressure, heart disease, and immune disorders. Other notable benefits of recreational therapy include improved physical health indicators such as bone density, heart rate, joint mobility, fine and gross motor coordination, balance, and strength, and it also reduces secondary disabilities such as decubitus ulcers and urinary tract infections (Peterson & Stumbo, 2000). Clients can experience any or all of these benefits depending on the recreational therapy program. Communication and social interactions are also benefits of rehabilitation therapies involving therapeutically designed activity. Injured patients often encounter feelings of isolation. Such feelings can be limiting to rehabilitation success, thus, positive experiences with peers and family during the engagement of leisure activity can often be very therapeutic.

Recreational therapy can also have a positive effect on a client's perception of locus of control. The principle of internal locus of control refers to an individual's perception of how responsible he or she is for his or her own behavior and for the outcomes of such behavior. Typically, individuals with a high internal locus of control take responsibility for their own decisions and for the consequences of their behaviors (which, in turn, enhances the individual's choice) (Peterson & Stumbo, 2000). Stimulating activity through recreational therapies increases cognitive insight and can positively affect locus of control and cognitive functioning, such as sequencing. Such activities can also help the individual organize his or her thought process with less effort because of the positive secondary effects.

Recreational therapy often takes place within the community, and is often utilized in more spontaneous ways than many other discipline-specific therapies. For example, the following observations can be made during an activity such as attending a movie:

- Money skills in the purchasing of tickets is information applicable to occupational therapy.
- Social interactions with strangers is applicable to cognitive choices in psychology and behavioral services.
- Nutritional choices at the snack counter for a diabetic is applicable to health promotion important for medical and nursing service professionals.
- Ability to access a seat away from the aisle is beneficial information for the physical therapist.
- On-task duration, stamina, attention span, and choice of movie are all useful activities and issues for the psychologist.

These are examples of information that could be communicated to the other treatment team professionals to help distinguish how effectively their discipline-specific therapies and modalities are being utilized by the client in a normalized or natural setting. A recreation therapy program design should include specific goals and criteria to ensure validity as a measurable therapy. The program/therapy needs to include formalized client assessment, statement of purpose, specific and measurable treatment goals, and general performance measures. These are components of effective accountability for any rehabilitation discipline to ensure that the process is systematic, logical, and relevant to the client's needs (Peterson & Stumbo, 2000).

Activity (therapy) selection is dependent on individual client needs or strengths and on predictive benefit. More important, the activity selection process must be compatible with client preferences, to help ensure "buy in" by that client. Assessing and addressing leisure history, past and present relationships, and successes are often factors that can make new leisure skills easier to attain and more acceptable via positive reinforcement. Helping the client establish positive relationships with others during activities can be beneficial, since such activities shift the focus away from the disability and onto the person. One example of this is a TBI (traumatic brain injury) client who consistently beats the staff at billiards because he is simply a good billiards player—not a disabled man who happens to be good at billiards. Plato once said "you can learn more about a man in an afternoon of play than in a lifetime of work." Recreational therapy applies this logic by treating the whole person and not just the disability.

A COMMUNITY INTEGRATION MODEL

The purpose of this section is threefold:

1. To outline the role of the recreational therapist as part of an interdisciplinary team in the neurorehabilitation process.
2. To describe in detail the specific goals of recreational therapy within a TBI community integration model.
3. To review the structure and components of the recreational therapy/community integration program at a hospital-based neurorehabilitation program.

A hospital-based community integration program designed for persons with severe TBI and resulting neurobehavioral disorders may include an inpatient, day treatment, and/or a residential program component. Such programs, which typically are staffed by therapeutic recreational professionals and other rehabilitation staff, are part of the greater multidisciplinary services. As part of a comprehensive/holistic rehabilitation milieu, the therapeutic recreation program is designed to address the four primary needs of a TBI patient. These include

- cognitive/emotional,
- psychological/spiritual,
- physical, and
- behavioral needs.

The primary goals of a therapeutic recreation service within a community integration program include the following:

- To increase self-initiated leisure and creative activity
- To reduce levels of agitation and aggressive behaviors
- To increase prevocational and vocational skills
- To increase cognitive and physical (motor coordination, etc.) functioning
- To provide real-life opportunities for application of newly acquired skills
- To assist with a smooth transition back into the community

Increasing Self-Initiated Leisure and Creative Activity

As described in Chapters 1 and 3 of this text, persons with severe TBI often present with executive functioning deficits, which includes a diminished ability to initiate appropriate, goal-directed, meaningful activity. As mentioned, one of the most devastating consequences of TBI is a patient's reduction in or total loss of meaningful activity in his or her life. As the patient's opportunity and ability to participate in leisure, pleasurable, and stress-reducing activities are significantly diminished, patients may experience depression and agitation (further isolating them from social and leisure opportunities). Through recreational therapies the patient is able to learn to participate in routine, purposeful, goal-directed activities that can be incrementally increased in complexity over time.

Reducing Levels of Agitation and Aggressive Behaviors

As noted in Chapter 3, it is physically impossible for the body to experience relaxation/calmness and anxiety/agitation (arousal) at the same time. Through recreational therapies, TBI patients are provided an environment and opportunity for naturally calming activities. During community-integration recreational therapies, staff promote patient awareness of body tension and emotional state while they are involved in the various emotionally relaxing/calming activities. Within these community settings and naturally relaxing situations, recreational and behavioral staff are able to discuss issues and concepts related to aggression and behavioral dysfunction with the patient. As part of the community-integration programming, staff coach the patient regarding (1) the application of physical- and emotional-control techniques during physically relaxing activities, (2) methods of increasing his or her anger and frustration threshold, and (3) generalization of various stress-coping strategies. Such concepts and therapeutic interactions occur on both an informal and formal basis. Thus, the recreational therapeutic milieu becomes a catalyst for staff and patients to address significant behavioral difficulties in a naturally calm, nonthreatening, and real-life environment.

Increasing Prevocational and Vocational Skills

Another devastating consequence of severe TBI is a person's inability to return to gainful employment (Buffington & Malec, 1997). As much of a person's self-image and self-esteem is determined by what a person does, the loss of vocational skills and ability due to cognitive, physical, and behavioral deficits can be catastrophic to the individual's emotional state and well-being. Unfortunately the loss of involvement in vocational and even leisure activity exacerbates the emotional and behavioral disturbances. Through recreational therapy, prevocational skill building and assessment can be conducted in an emotionally and physically safe environment. During the community-integration activities, the interdisciplinary team can assist patients in regaining skills in cognitive (planning, problem solving, sequencing, attention, concentration, and mental flexibility), emotional/psychological (anger management, emotions regulation, and anxiety reduction) and physical abilities.

Increasing Cognitive and Physical Functioning

As many neurobehaviorally disordered TBI patients are often resistant to participating in traditional rehabilitation therapies provided through traditional modalities (such as physical, occupational, and cognitive therapy), recreational therapy activities provide an environment conducive to positive nonconfrontational therapist/patient interaction. Patients tend to be in a more relaxed and nondefensive physical, mental, and emotional state during these art therapies and, thus, are much more willing (even unknowingly so) to participate in activities that improve cognitive, psychomotor, and other physical functioning. For example, community activity planning is a useful tool in enhancing learning and problem-solving abilities, which are common cognitive deficits and are contributors to neurobehavioral dysfunction in persons with TBI. In coordination with the physical and occupational therapists, neuropsychologist, and physician, the recreational therapist can design and implement community-integration activities that directly address the discipline-specific goals. For a patient with psychomotor difficulties, for example, an individual plan could be designed that incrementally increases the difficulty of a recreational task over each session or activity. Also, as recreational therapeutic activities can range from very basic to complex (both cognitively and physically), specific therapies can be introduced according to the patient's individual abilities and needs.

During daily patient rounds and weekly treatment-plan meetings, the recreational therapist coordinates with the psychologist, the physical and occupational therapist, and other rehabilitation team members to develop a community-integration treatment plan.

Providing Real-Life Opportunities for Application of Newly Acquired Skills

Although the TBI patient is able to learn and apply various skills from other rehabilitation disciplines in a well-structured and controlled environment, the recreational therapy services and community-integration program provide the patient an opportunity to apply these skills to real-life situations in the community. The community-based activities provide a chance for assessment of the patient's ability to apply and generalize skills and knowledge obtained in more "traditional" rehabilitation settings while managing the risk of harm to self and others. Research with this patient population continues to demonstrate the importance and efficacy of the use of supportive work trials and other real-life activities as part of the rehabilitation process.

Often, when a patient comes from a rehabilitation setting, it is structured for higher levels of safety, stimulation is controlled, and staff is available for more immediate attention and assistance.

In a community setting, more coping strategies are required to accomplish tasks we take for granted (for example, waiting in line, interaction with service personnel, and traffic patterns). Social cues are not understood and the result can impede community transition. Exposure and decentralization to these stressful situations along with individual prompting can lessen the level of anxiety in the community setting and make cognitive decision making more productive.

An example might be returning an item to a store. Generally, most retailers have lenient policies on returns or refunds. A patient might only require a refund but store policy allows store credit only; the ongoing situation might be exacerbated by a rude employee. To a patient with impulse control, the situation can become volatile quickly. A plan for this type of community activity requires a sequential action that the patient understands and has contingencies that they can accept without behavioral outbursts. Generally, prior planning prevents these events.

THE ROLE OF THE HOSPITAL-BASED RECREATIONAL THERAPIST

The hospital-based recreational therapist (RT) is trained to coordinate the hospital or rehabilitation service community integration program and typically supervises the recreational program staff. The RT and community integration program are often part of the hospital's neurobehavioral services department, which may include neuropsychology, psychology, behavioral therapy, recreational therapy, and spiritual counseling staff. The RT is typically supervised directly by a director of neurobehavioral services or the rehabilitation department supervisor. As the community-integration program coordinator, the RT is a key member of the hospital's rehabilitation treatment team, which provides clinical direction to the rehabilitation program and oversees the development and implementation of the patient's treatment plan. In addition, the RT attends all rehabilitation coordination meetings, treatment-planning meetings, and patient rounds. Through this system and structure, the RT is able to effectively communicate and coordinate with all other disciplines and therapists on a daily basis. The organizational structure of the recreational therapy service establishes a means for clear interface between the goals and services established/provided by the various rehabilitation disciplines and the goals of the community integration program. Various coordination and clinical meetings held throughout the week ensure consistency of patient services and a near seamless system through four phases of the neurobehavioral rehabilitation process (see Figure 6.1).

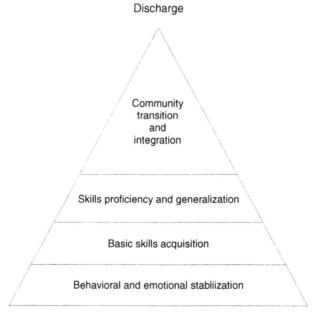

FIGURE 6.1. Four-stage hospital-based rehabilitation model. (*Source:* Murrey et al., 2004)

THE HOSPITAL-BASED
COMMUNITY-INTEGRATION PROGRAM

The hospital-based community-integration program includes a multicomponent system focusing directly on the patient's primary neurorehabilitation goals, which are established by the entire treatment team. Each activity should be designed to help patients address their primary treatment needs and move them through the four phases of the rehabilitation process discussed previously. The following section describes the primary components of a community-integration program.

Leisure and Recreational Skills Therapy

As previously discussed, leisure and recreational planning skills are often diminished and/or completely lost after brain injury. Two main components of recreational therapy are (1) to provide opportunities for the patient to participate in leisure/recreational activities during the time that he or she is a patient in the hospital or other rehabilitation program, and (2) to help the patient develop skills in seeking out recreational or leisure opportunities, developing and implementing a plan for such activities, and self-initiating to participate in such activities.

Though these tasks may seem very simple to a person without a brain injury, to a patient who has a variety of cognitive or executive and physical impairments, they can be overwhelming and nearly impossible tasks to complete. For example, patients may be able to state what they would like to do but may not be able to self-initiate even the simplest behaviors to begin the process or activity. Through progressive treatment with a recreational therapist the patient begins to relearn the skills necessary to break down planning of activities and tasks into simple and workable components, and begins to develop and review opportunities for leisure activities. These can be as simple as organizing a group for a card game to more complex tasks as an extended trip to a big city.

Troubleshooting or problem solving during community-based activities is also a primary therapeutic issue in recreational therapy. For example, helping patients find their way around town, use public transportation, or locate appropriate persons to find assistance if they become lost are all complex tasks that can be addressed in therapy. Through the community-based recreational and leisure activities, the recreational therapist and recreational therapy program staff can provide real-life tests and application opportunities of skills and functions being addressed by other disciplines within the hospital setting. Examples of this include assessment of mobility and ambulation and other physical functioning by the physical and occupational therapist while the patient participates in leisure activities in the community; assessment of planning and problem solving and other cognitive skills by the speech therapist and neuropsychologist; and assessment of anger and frustration management and other behavioral issues by the behavioral therapist and psychologist.

Budgeting Skills

Since most patients who have suffered a severe traumatic brain injury will need to learn to live off of a reduced or fixed income, money management and budget planning are critical skills for these patients. However, as previously discussed, many patients with a severe brain injury also present with poor impulse control and behavioral disinhibition, which can include impulse buying and spending. Such behaviors, combined with limited funds, quickly result in patients having no funds in a very short period of time, which leads to further frustration, agitation, and physical aggression. Lack of funds may often lead to very limited leisure and recreational opportunities. Recreational therapy, in cooperation with other therapies (speech, occupational, etc.) can help patients learn and apply such skills as budget planning and spending prioritization. During community-based treatments and activities, the recreational therapist provides the patients with cues and skill-building techniques regarding purchase choices and priorities, and cues them back to their preestablished budget/spending plan.

Community Integration Assessment and Therapy

The recreational therapist plays a critical role in assessing the patient's abilities and deficits while in the community. Such assessments provide members of the treatment team and other disciplines important information on the patient's readiness to return to the community and in what specific areas the patient will need continued support or assistance. This comprehensive community integration assessment includes an evaluation of a patient's applied cognitive abilities (problem solving, decision making, processing speed, memory, etc.), practical observed physical functioning (mobility, balance, fine and gross motor skills, etc.), and behavioral skills (anger and impulse control, socially appropriate interactions, etc.). The professionals coordinate each of these discipline-specific issues and treatments and provide them with a list of specific areas of concern. In addition, the team members can develop, with the recreational therapist, observation and other assessment tools to document strengths, abilities, and weaknesses or deficits in target areas to be used during community activities. The community-integration services and program can be the capstone of a multidiscipline area and holistic rehabilitation program since it provides an opportunity to observe and assess a patient (and provide therapeutic intervention) within a multitude of real-life situations and environments. The list of situations are limitless and include such activities as shopping, playing sports, interacting with friends and family, or participating as a volunteer or as an employee in a supportive work trial.

Aquatic Therapy and Exercise Program

Use of exercise and swimming are wonderful therapeutic and health-building opportunities often overlooked in many rehabilitation programs. However, due to physical changes and disabilities, higher fatigue, and general decreased physical activity level, the brain-injured person is even more prone to obesity and general muscle atrophy. Thus, establishing an individualized, structured, and scheduled exercise program soon after the brain injury and prior to the person returning to the community is critical. Recreational therapists typically have education and background in exercise training and health promotion. Thus, recreational therapists are a logical choice to direct the development and implementation of specialized exercise programming (in coordination with the physical therapists and medical/nursing staff). In addition, the use of water is a method of facilitating less painful and more enjoyable exercise, thus range of motion and strength building, can be employed by the treatment team. Formal or informal aquatic therapy programs can be facilitated by the recreational therapist, again, in conjunction with the physical therapist, physician, nurses, and other such team members. Even though most hospitals and/or rehabilitation programs do not have an on-site pool, recreational therapists can often locate facilities where these therapies can take place. Possibilities may include high schools, colleges, YMCAs, or private health clubs with swimming facilities. Such facilities or organizations are often willing to allow use of pools during low-attendance times or times that they are not being used for minimal to no cost to the patient. In addition, community organizations are often willing to provide funding for patients to use such facilities.

Vocational Retraining Program

Though it may seem somewhat of an oxymoron, the recreational therapist (perhaps better called the community-integration coordinator) can also serve as a vocational therapy/program coordinator. Equally devastating as the loss of opportunities to participate in leisure and recreational activities is the loss of ability or opportunity to work. For most people, a person's job defines who they are and is a primary source of self-esteem. Unfortunately, the vast majority of persons who have suffered a severe traumatic brain injury do not return to any form of work, let alone competitive employment with the opportunity to advance and progress within a particular vocation. However, by focusing on vocational and prevocational skills and retraining early in the rehabilitation process, potential for return to some form of work (even if that is as a volunteer or within a supportive work program) is significantly increased. In consultation with the treatment team, the recreational therapist can develop both individual and group work-trial programs and opportunities. These can include both on-site and community-based volunteer or paid work. These can also be coordinated through the state's vocational rehabilitation services or coordinated directly with various employers and organizations in the community. In the hospital-based rehabilitation program, assessments for readiness and prevocational skills as well as adaptive equipment needs should be conducted by various members of the multidisciplinary team including the physical, behavioral, speech, and occupational therapists as well as the neuropsychologist and physician. Simple evaluations (such as the example provided in Figure 6.2) can be developed and used by recreational therapy staff or even

COMMUNITY/VOCATIONAL SKILLS ASSESSMENT FORM

Patient Name: _____ Location: _____ Task(s): _____

Skill	Always	Usually	Needs Improve-ment
Prompt			
Dresses appropriately			
Polite to supervisors/staff			
Polite to co-workers/peers			
Follows instructions			
Remains on task during assigned time			
Fully completes task			
Seeks another appropriate activity when assigned task is complete			
Uses special accommodations/ resources when needed			
Is able to orient to surroundings consistently			
Recommendations:			

Staff Signature _____

Date: _____

Name
Med rec #:

Birth date:
Gender:
Program/unit:

FIGURE 6.2. Community/vocation skills assessment form.

work-trial supervisors to document the patient's strengths, weaknesses, and progress during each work trial or activity.

Art Therapy Program

Depending on the skills and interests of the recreational therapist or other rehabilitation staff, an art therapy program could be developed. As outlined in more detail in Chapter 3, the goals of art therapy in a hospital-based rehabilitation program for TBI persons include the following:

• To increase self-initiated leisure and creative activity.
• To provide an alternative modality for assessments to better understand the patient.
• To promote expression of emotions and thoughts not often expressed in a socially appropriate manner.
• To increase cognitive and physical (fine motor coordination) functioning.
• To reduce levels of agitation and aggressive behaviors.

Horticultural Therapy Program

A horticultural therapy program, on either a small or large scale, can be a wonderful modality for providing multidiscipline therapies and assessment. The recreational therapist can be a key player in the development, implementation, and coordination of such a program along with other professionals including physical, occupational, and behavioral therapists. Goals and approaches of horticultural therapy are discussed in more detail in Chapter 2 of this text.

Obviously, recreational therapy is only one piece of the interdisciplinary, holistic rehabilitation program available to a hospital-based program. As such, it is difficult to fully evaluate the contributions of recreational therapy program in isolation from the other therapeutic services. However, behavioral data evaluations and studies have demonstrated promising clinical and postdischarge outcome findings. Specifically, since the formal introduction of various components of community integration into hospital-based therapy programs, the number of required physical restraints and seclusions of patients due to aggressive behaviors has declined significantly. In addition, postdischarge outcome studies of patients up to three years following discharge continue to show patients maintaining their behavioral stability and gains over time with many still applying their skills, knowledge, and interest in recreational, vocational, and horticultural activities in the community. Such findings are consistent with research that has been conducted on similar disability groups. However, continued and more in-depth research on the benefits of recreational and community-integration therapy for persons with traumatic brain injury and associated neurobehavioral disorders is needed.

TRAINING AND EDUCATIONAL PROGRAMS

Several colleges and universities have bachelor's and master's degree programs in therapeutic recreation. Some of these are specifically approved by a therapeutic recreation certifying agency or board as meeting their academic requirements. A comprehensive listing of these institutions is available at the following Web site: <http://www.recreationtherapy.com/trcollg.htm>.

Memberships and Board Certification

Organizations in the United States that currently promote the discipline of therapeutic recreation include:

- National Therapeutic Recreation Society (NTRS)
- American Therapeutic Recreation Association (ATRA)
- National Recreation and Park Association (NRPA)
- National Council for Therapeutic Recreation Certification (NCTRC)

These organizations have defined the standards for the certification of professionals and the promotion of this discipline.

Information regarding professional organizations/membership services in therapeutic recreation can be obtained through the following sources:

1. The American Therapeutic Recreation Association (ATRA) at <www.atra-tr.org> or by writing to ATRA, 1414 Prince Street,

Suite 204, Alexandria, Virginia 22314. Telephone 703-683-9420; Fax 703-683-9431.
2. National Recreation and Park Association (NRPA) at <www.nrpa.org> or by writing to 22377 Belmont Ridge Road, Ashburn, Virginia 20148. Telephone 703-858-0784; Fax 703-858-0794.

Information relating to board certification can be obtained by contacting:

1. The National Council for Therapeutic Recreation Certification (NCTRC) at <www.nctrc.org> or by writing to 7 Elmwood Drive, New City, New York 10956. Telephone 845-639-1439; Fax: 845-639-1471.

   The NCTRC provides a special certification to recreational therapists who have completed training in an NCTRC-approved program or other program that meets their requirements. Persons receiving this certification become Certified Therapeutic Recreational Specialists (CTRS).
2. The National Recreation and Park Association (NRPA) at <www.nrpa.org> or by writing to 22377 Belmont Ridge Road, Ashburn, Virginia 20148-4501. Telephone 703-858-0784; Fax 703-858-0794

   The NRPA provides a general certification for recreational and leisure professionals. A person completing this certification becomes a certified leisure professional.

BIBLIOGRAPHY

Buffington, A. L., & Malec, J. F. (1997). The vocational rehabilitation continuum: Maximizing outcomes through bridging the gap from hospital to community-based services. *The Journal of Head Trauma Rehabilitation, 12*(5), 1-13.

Bullock, C. C., & Mahon, M. J. (2001). *Introduction to Recreation Services for People with Disabilities: A Person-Centered Approach.* Champaign, IL: Sagamore Publishing.

Goldstein, R. C., & Levin, H. S. (1995). Neurobehavioral outcome of traumatic brain injury: Coma, the vegetative state, and the minimally responsive state. *The Journal of Head Trauma Rehabilitation, 10*(1), 57-73.

Grace, J., Stout, J. C., & Malloy, P. F. (1999). Assessing frontal lobe behavioral syndromes with the frontal lobe personality scale. *Psychological Assessment Resources, 6*(3), 269-284.

Grafman, J., Sirigu, A., Spector, L., & Hendler, J. (1993). Damage to the prefrontal cortex leads to decomposition of structured event complexes. *The Journal of Head Trauma Rehabilitation, 8*(1), 73-87.

Hart, T., & Jacobs, H. E. (1993). Rehabilitation and management of behavioral disturbances following frontal lobe injury. *The Journal of Head Trauma Rehabilitation, 8*(1), 1-12.

Jacobs, H. E. (1997). The clubhouse: Addressing work-related behavioral challenges through a supportive social community. *The Journal of Head Trauma Rehabilitation, 12*(5), 14-27.

Jacobson, E. (1938). *Progressive Relaxation.* Chicago: University of Chicago Press.

Jacobson, E. (1948). *You Must Relax: A Practical Method for Reducing the Strains of Modern Living.* New York: McGraw-Hill Book Company, Inc.

Lezak, M. D. (1993). Newer contributions to the neuropsychological assessment of executive functions. *The Journal of Trauma Rehabilitation, 8*(1), 24-31.

Murrey, G. J., Helgeson, S. R., Courtney, C. T. , & Starzinski, D. T. (1998). State-coordinated services for traumatic brain injury survivors: Toward a model delivery system. *The Journal of Head Trauma Rehabilitation, 13*(6), 72-81.

Murrey, G. J., Starzinski, D. T., and LeBlanc, A. J. (2004). Base Rates of Traumatic Brain Injury History in Adults Admitted to State Psychiatric Hospitals: A 3-Year Study. *Rehabilitation Psychology, 49*(3): 259-261.

Peterson, C. A., & Stumbo, N. J. (2000). *Therapeutic recreation program design. Principles and Procedures.* Enumclaw, WA: Idyll Arbor.

Prigatano, G. P. (1999a). *Principles of Neuropsychological Rehabilitation.* New York: Oxford University Press.

Prigatano, G. P. (1999b). *Principles of Neuropsychological Rehabilitation.* New York: Oxford University Press.

Rosenthal, M., Christensen, B. K., & Ross, T. P. (1998). Depression following traumatic brain injury. *Archives of Physical Medicine & Rehabilitation, 79,* 90-103.

Sander, A. M., Kreutzer, J. S., & Fernandez, C. C. (1997). Neurobehavioral functioning, substance abuse, and employment after brain injury: Implications for vocational rehabilitation. *The Journal of Head Trauma Rehabilitation, 12*(5), 28-41.

Sohlberg, M. M., Mateer, C. A., & Stuss, D. T. (1993). Contemporary approaches to the management of executive control dysfunction. *The Journal of Head Trauma Rehabilitation, 8*(1), 45-58.

Trudel, T. M., Tyron, W. W., & Purdum, C. M. (1998). Awareness of disability and and long-term outcome after traumatic brain injury. *Rehabilitation Psychology, 43*(4), 267-281.

Varney, N. R., & Menefee, L. (1993). Psychosocial and executive deficits following closed head injury: Implications for orbital frontal cortex. *The Journal of Head Trauma Rehabilitation, 8*(1), 32-44.

Wehman, P. H., West, M. D., Kregel, J., Sherron, P., & Kreutzer, J. S. (1995). Return to work for persons with severe traumatic brain injury: A data-based approach to program development. *The Journal of Head Trauma Rehabilitation, 10*(1), 27-39.

Wolpe, J. (1969). *The Practice of Behavior Therapy.* New York: Pergamon Press.

Chapter 7

Chemical-Dependency Treatment with Traumatic Brain-Injured Clients

Duane A. Reynolds
Gregory J. Murrey

INTRODUCTION AND OVERVIEW

The use of legal and illegal mood-altering substances places individuals at greater risk for motor vehicle accidents, assaults/violent behavior, sports and recreation injuries, and falls. The co-occurring use of alcohol and drugs after brain injury has also been well documented (Bogner et al., 1997; Corrigan et al., 1999; Corrigan et al., 1995; Kreutzer et al., 1996). More than 1.5 million injuries occur each year in the United States, and a significant number of these accidents involve the use of alcohol and drugs. Alcohol is the primary substance abused in the United States since it is legal and easy to purchase. Sixty-six percent of mild brain injuries and 73 percent of moderate injuries involve the use of alcohol. Equally concerning is that 30 to 50 percent of these persons who suffer a TBI (traumatic brain injury) return to alcohol abuse after medical recovery.

Although chemical-dependency recovery treatment programs exist that specifically treat clients with traumatic brain injury, the majority of TBI clients with chemical-dependency (CD) issues are mainstreamed into traditional chemical dependency programs with other clients from their community. Certainly, some strong arguments can be made for not removing TBI clients from their community, such as the proximity of their medical team or family and the cost of inpatient treatment (which often make such community-based services the first choice). Unfortunately, the traditional community-based CD program may not be the most appropriate for TBI clients who have attentional, processing, or other cognitive impairments. Brain-injured clients often feel left behind while trying to adapt to a cognitive modality that does not take into consideration their postinjury learning deficits (Karol, 2003). Frequently, in mainstream CD programs, TBI clients are underdiagnosed or identified only after they have failed several treatment experiences. In the meantime, their cognitive abilities continue to decrease due to the continued abuse of alcohol and drugs.

Traditional cognitive abstinence-based programming may not be flexible enough to provide for a beneficial experience for a cognitively impaired TBI client. The Americans with Disabilities Act (ADA) gives some direction to treatment programs that have clients with physical or mental impairments that substantially limit one or more major life activities. Clients who have a record of such an impairment through testing and history and are regarded as having an impairment are protected by this law. Impairment in major life activities or essential functions may include reduced ability in such areas as performing personal care or manual tasks, walking, vision, hearing, speaking, breathing, thinking, learning, and/or working. The ADA states that treatment programs cannot require people to attend special programs but must, at minimum, make reasonable accommodation in the existing programming. Programs, thus, need to remove barriers to effective communication and learning for such clients, and all new construction must be barrier free and have annual reviews to develop readily achievable goals for ongoing accommodation.

Treatment programs should be prepared to mainstream their clients with different learning styles and abilities by making reasonable modifications to policy and procedures by furnishing aids for effective communication and by working to remove barriers to participation. If necessary, alternative services should be offered, such as brain injury support groups or therapies. Fortunately, the majority of TBIs are mild, but even mild injuries can result in the need for major compensatory adjustments or accommodations.

Brain injuries of any level can result in any or all of the following impairments:

• Disinhibition/decreased impulse control
• Increased anger/aggression

- Social inappropriateness
- Altered self-image
- Decreased visual motor skills
- Memory impairment short and long term
- Poor concentration or difficulty with abstract concepts resulting in appearing to be disinterested or uninvolved
- Lack of strength and endurance
- Sensory deficits—smell, taste, touch, and vision
- Sexual disinterest or preoccupation/disinhibition
- Impaired executive functioning (the ability to plan, prioritize, organize, set goals, execute strategies, and monitor behavior)

Thus, CD programs that treat persons with TBI need to train staff on how to accommodate such clients and cognitive deficits.

TREATMENT OF PATIENTS WITH EXECUTIVE DYSFUNCTION: CLINICAL CONSIDERATIONS

Many persons who have suffered severe traumatic injury to the frontal temporal regions of the brain present with significant deficits in executive functioning and associated neurobehavioral disorders (Grace, Stout, & Malloy, 1999; Prigatano, 1999; Sohlberg, Matteer, & Struss, 1993; Trudel, Tyron, & Purdum, 1998). As discussed in Chapter 1 of this text, these neurobehavioral disorders can include disturbances in initiation, impulse control, problem solving, and frustration tolerance (Goldstein and Levin, 1995; Prigatano, 1999). Such deficits can further exacerbate the individual's preexisting chemical-dependency issues and/or increase risk for chemical abuse (Delmonico, Hanley-Peterson, & Englander, 1998). Although a few recent articles have been published on screening for substance abuse in persons with a TBI (e.g., Arenth, Bogner, Corrigan, & Schmidt, 2001) and on the use of traditional substance abuse treatment models with this unique patient population (e.g., Kramer & Hoisington, 1992), little, if any, literature discusses specialized programming for the TBI patient with executive control deficits.

Overview of the Executive Functions

The executive functions have been tied to the frontal lobes of the brain, which, in essence, act as an executor or overseer of all other areas of the brain. The frontal cortex oversees the thoughts, emotions, and behaviors of an individual, receiving messages and feedback and sending commands via the neuropathways throughout the brain. Due to the structure of the skull and location of the frontal lobes of the brain, the frontal and temporal lobes are very susceptible to damage, particularly during motor vehicle accidents. Damage to the dorsal prefrontal regions and the orbital frontal regions of the frontal lobes can result in a negative and positive symptom presentation, respectively. It is not uncommon for a brain-injured person to present with adynamia (inability to initiate behavior) and perseveration or impulsivity (inability to stop or inhibit behaviors). Thus, the person could have difficulty starting a behavior but also may have difficulty stopping the activity or behavior once initiated. A primary executive function disorder that is often not well understood by clinicians, counselors, or even medical professionals is anosognosia ("anos" meaning self and "agnosia" meaning inability to recognize), which refers to the lack of awareness of deficit due to frontal lobe damage and corresponding executive dysfunction. It is important for the counselor to understand the difference between anosognosia (lack of awareness of deficit) and denial. Specifically, anosognosia is a result of an actual neurocognitive disorder due to a neurological trauma, whereas denial is a psychological construct that is psychiatric in nature and anxiety based.

Treatment Considerations for the TBI Patient with Executive Dysfunction

Considering that executive dysfunction can have a significant effect on patients with brain injury and corresponding chemical-abuse issues, clinicians need to be cognizant of a variety of treatment issues with this particular population. Some of the other specific clinical issues that need to be considered when developing a chemical-dependency treatment plan or program for persons with TBI and associated executive dysfunction are outlined as follows:

- *Diminished emotional regulation and labile mood.* Due to changes in the neurochemicals of the brain, TBI patients may be highly prone to depression, agitation, low frustration tolerance, and rapid mood swings.
- *Diminished speed of information processing, attention and concentration, and mental flexibility.* TBI patients may have difficulty keeping up with other patients in group settings. Attention span, speed of processing, and comprehension/processing of verbally presented information may be significantly reduced, making it difficult for them to fully benefit from traditional substance abuse treatment modalities.
- *Diminished memory functions.* TBI patients typically present with diminished ability to store, recall, and apply new information. They are also very sensitive to high levels of stimuli, which can adversely affect their already diminished memory capacity. Such deficits can be very problematic within a traditional substance-abuse therapy program that seeks to educate patients by providing them with increased knowledge regarding the chemical abuse.
- *Diminished insight and self-monitoring.* As previously discussed, patients with executive dyscontrol often suffer from anosognosia as well as diminished ability to monitor one's own behaviors. Such deficits can be very problematic since CD treatment is insight-oriented.
- *Diminished impulse/behavioral control.* TBI patients with executive dysfunction often present with increased impulsivity and diminished capacity to inhibit inappropriate behaviors. Such behaviors obviously are in direct conflict with the behaviors that the CD counselor is trying to promote—that is, taking responsibility and control over the addictive behaviors. Such deficits only exacerbate the already problematic abuse lifestyle.

TRADITIONAL TREATMENT APPROACHES

Mainstream or traditional CD treatment programs may typically base their therapeutic approach on one of several orientations. Some of these traditional therapy models include insight-oriented treatment, skill-building treatment approaches, and traditional behavior treatments.

Insight-Oriented Treatment

In insight-oriented treatment, the primary goal is to build personal insight by providing information and promoting introspection by exploring consequences such as working on the twelve steps of Alcoholics Anonymous, teaching the disease concept, and having clients read a variety of self-help educational books while completing standard assignments. The philosophy behind this approach is that information changes ways of thinking, and changes in thinking lead to changes in behavior. However, TBI clients may have difficulty expressing their thoughts or gaining insight into their deficits (due to the anosognosia). In addition, slowed mental processing can be frustrating for clients when they cannot arrive at an answer as quickly as nonimpaired clients. They may want to answer but need more time to respond, thus creating frustration in such situations. Some disabled clients may also not be able to change their thoughts or gain insight due to cognitive deficits resulting from the injury. Surprisingly, brain-injured clients may not change their behavior even if they do gain insight or increased awareness of the negative effects of their behaviors because of their executive dysfunctions.

Skill-Building Treatment

The skill-building technique seeks to teach alternative behaviors and skills. The theory behind this treatment approach is that new and more effective skills and behaviors will replace old, ineffective behaviors or provide the client with additional behavioral options. However, disability issues for TBI clients may result in great difficulty learning new skills. They may perseverate their old ineffective behavior and forget to implement the new skills when the situation warrants, or they may even distort the new skill.

Traditional Behavioral Treatment

The behavioral technique seeks to manipulate a client's behavior via the use of consequences and reinforcers—the theory being that the client will experience behavioral change due to such consequences. However, disability issues for the TBI client may result in the client forgetting the new behavior, forgetting the consequences, perseverating old behavior styles, or rebelling against the consequences; alternatively, the consequences may be too weak to change behaviors. In some cases the client often does not act in his or her own best interest and, thus, traditional behavioral approaches are often not effective (or may even be contraindicated) with TBI clients.

A Model of Treatment for Clients with TBI and Related Cognitive Disability

Accurate assessment of the client with chemical abuse history is a critical step. An assessment needs to determine how aware the client is of cognitive deficits and abuse problems. If the client lacks awareness or has only very limited awareness of the existence of an alcohol or drug problem, he or she will likely be unable to recognize deficits and have difficulty internalizing problems associated with actual or potential consequences associated with the substance use. If insight is minimal or lacking (due to anosognosia secondary to the TBI), external structure and a structured environment that limits exposure to triggers and cues in the patient's environment will be necessary. Typically, this would include a residential program offering twenty-four-hour supervision.

If clients have some intellectual awareness and insight into a substance-abuse problem, they may be able to recognize past problems but might not be able to predict when or how they will effectively avoid high-risk situations in the future. In such instances, they may not be able to effectively apply newly learned skills when they are needed. Thus, they may need ongoing external cueing to implement strategies to avoid further substance abuse. The client could be taught standard responses to future events with the use of memory aids, role-playing, and external cues. In addition, a partial-day program offering up to seven hours of programming per day may be adequate for such clients.

If clients have an emergent awareness of their deficits and abuse problems, they are reaching a point at which they can recognize problems associated with their deficits as they occur. They can typically use treatment strategies but may need help anticipating when they will be needed and how best to implement these strategies and skills.

A primary approach to assist such clients is to develop "stop, think, and act" strategies, which are similar to anger de-escalation techniques. In addition, an appropriate outpatient CD treatment program with four or more hours of programming would be appropriate and likely meet the needs for this type of TBI client.

If a client has anticipatory awareness, he or she can typically anticipate future problems and respond by giving cues utilizing "stop, think, and act" strategies independently. Weekly outpatient groups or individual therapy is recommended and usually is sufficient to meet this client's needs.

Many clients are placed in the "least-restrictive" treatment setting, namely outpatient or day treatment programs, but due to cognitive and behavioral deficits in TBI clients, residential treatment or day treatment services with a structured living option may be necessary. Accurate assessment and the appropriate level of care greatly improve client outcome. Fatigue factors can also influence a given client's ability to participate. Consideration should be given to attendance two to three times per week for an extended period of time as opposed to requiring full-day attendance five days a week.

Clinicians need to be fully knowledgeable of the client's history, which is available in medical charts and reports as well as any disability-related testing reports. A neuropsychologist may need to evaluate the client to determine current cognitive functioning levels, and a psychiatrist may need to evaluate the client for medication management needs. Brain injury can exacerbate or exaggerate preinjury personality characteristics and chemical-abuse issues. Frequently, clients appear to have co-occurring disorders, but these need to be professionally evaluated (not assumed to exist) and treated. Prescribed medications may not be at therapeutic levels if the client is not taking the medications as prescribed. The client should be given time to "level off" and adjust to a normal routine. This also gives the therapist time to gather information and develop individualized treatment strategies.

Treatment Approach Comparison

Traditional treatment takes a cognitive- and/or reality-based approach; it is client centered, usually insight oriented, and abstinence based. The expectations are established and the treatment milieu developed to accommodate a certain number of clients. Group sizes and daily activities are designed for a certain level of functioning, and adjunctive therapies such as recreation, art, and music therapies may not be available. Using the twelve steps of Alcoholics Anonymous, which requires intact memory and the ability to sequence, prioritize, and plan, can be difficult for TBI clients unless accommodations are made.

Disability strategies are a type of motivational therapy that relies on motivational-interviewing techniques to support the client. Disability strategies are also client centered with the focus of treatment being on relapse containment. It is basically a "harm-reduction" model as opposed to an "abstinence-based" model. Insight is not as important as lifestyle analysis. Treatment focuses on the cues and triggers in the client's environment, the client's beliefs about substance use, and beliefs about the client's disability and his or her awareness of deficits. Using this strategy, the therapist also must ascertain the client's preferred learning style and what accommodations need to be made so that he or she can progress in treatment. For example, clients with word-recognition deficits would need individual verbal therapy sessions and tape-recorded assignments as opposed to worksheets and written assignments.

Disability strategies place more emphasis on individual client and private family sessions and focus on multidisciplinary integration. For this model to work effectively with the TBI client, the various professionals must be diligent in communicating together so that all are working toward the same treatment goals. Disability strategies take a supportive role with the client and are more suggestive than directive. In this treatment, motivational interviewing techniques can be useful. The therapist works with the client to examine a variety of reasons/causes/motivations for substance abuse and strives to identify limitations, develop compensatory skills, and help the client accept such limitations.

Traditional treatment focuses on group therapy and, if offered, family groups. However, large groups can have multiple distractions and multiple verbal and nonverbal interactions. For example, a client with deficits in attention, language comprehension, or sequencing may become distracted and confused, resulting in a withdrawal from the therapeutic process.

This treatment model is also based on the medical model and can be confrontational and direct. Using this model, such statements as "I know what's best for you," may be communicated or at least implied. This model is based more on the disease concept and on breaking denial. Also, some clients with TBI have organic insightlessness rather than denial. Confrontation only serves to demoralize the person and increase defensiveness.

TWO MODELS OF DISABILITY:
MEDICAL VERSUS INTERACTIONAL MODEL

The medical model assumes that a disability is a deficiency or abnormality. The disability is perceived as negative and the disability resides in the individual. The remedy for a disability-related problem is a cure or normalization of the individual and the agent of the remedy is the professional. Many people when hospitalized experience the "cure approach." The treatments are scheduled, tests are conducted, and progress is rated according to predetermined standards. In this model, clients are seldom asked for active involvement in the process.

In contrast, the interactional model assumes the disability is a difference or change rather than a "deficiency." In this model, being disabled is in itself neutral and the disability is derived from the interactions between the individual and society. According to this model, the remedy for a disability-related problem is a change in the interaction between the individual and society. The agent of such change can be the individual, the advocate, or anyone who can change these interactions. For example, a young woman with a history of TBI and chemical dependency was employed in a sheltered job situation and was very dependable. She enjoyed working on the food-serving line and interacting with customers. Due to being trustworthy and dependable, she was placed in the back room to cut cardboard boxes for recycling. She could perform the task without any danger of self-injury and could work independently. However, she experienced a decrease in job satisfaction due to the lack of contact with others, which was something she valued highly. The change agent was her case manager who, after much negotiation with the employer, was able to return her to her previous assignment with some minor accommodations.

Abstinence versus Harm Reduction

For the TBI client, a strong case can be made for use of an abstinence-based model of treatment. Some reasons for the use of this particular model include the following:

- The effects of alcohol and drugs can contribute to greater impairment of cognitive and motor skills.
- Dangerous interactions can occur between prescription medications and nonprescription drugs and alcohol.
- The continued use of alcohol and drugs increases the likelihood of seizures or other medical complications.
- TBI clients experience increased sensitivity to the effects of alcohol and drugs.

Harm reduction (a key focus of the abstinence model) assumes that few will remain totally abstinent forever; however, with effort and appropriate structure or supervision, improvement can be made. If a client does relapse, it is more important to try to stop the episode as soon as possible and prevent further harm from occurring. To remain isolated or to be fearful of potential consequences may prevent clients from telling others about the event, which further prevents them from receiving assistance when they are in need of it most.

EDUCATIONAL STRATEGIES

Group Therapy

For the TBI client, sessions (other than recreational therapy or activity sessions) should be a maximum of forty-five minutes in length with no less than forty-five minutes between sessions. A combination of interactive and didactic lecture or topic-focused sessions may be used. All sessions should limit the amount of information covered. Clients with attention problems, physical pain, or memory deficits will not benefit from lengthy sessions. Groups should be limited to six to eight clients with adequate space for extra room between chairs to reduce the amount of external stimuli or noise encountered by the client. In addition, such extra spacing between clients is especially advised for TBI clients with a history of physical aggression.

Individual Sessions

Individual sessions should not be more than twenty minutes in length and provided multiple times per week or per day. Typically, more can be accomplished for this clientele with three twenty-minute sessions than a single one-hour session. Clinicians should sit close to the client, and give their full attention. Clinicians should also encourage the client to use short sentences and stop when the thought is completed. Clients with severe communication deficits will require the clinician's complete attention and patience. In extreme cases, communication may need to be conducted one word at a time. The client may need to write his or her responses if a significant aphasia is present.

Stimulus and Distractor Reduction Techniques

Sessions should be conducted in an environment free from distractions. The more clutter allowed in the office or therapy space, the more distracting it is for clients with impulse-control issues and attention deficits. Such things as wall decorations should be limited and soft lighting with, ideally, no windows within the therapy setting is recommended.

Other Environmental and Behavioral Modification Strategies

Poster boards, signs, and symbols can be used to provide external cueing to assist the client in implementing compensatory strategies. A sign that reminds clients to shower daily can be used to remind those with a decreased sense of smell. Additional signs and reminders to take medications on time can increase medication compliance. A "practice anger control" sign reminds clients to focus on new skills learned to reduce anger flare-ups and a "keep your room clean" sign can result in fewer misplaced items. Such signs can be used in conjunction with teaching strategies, such as the following anger-reduction cue:

ANGER

Anticipate the situations that trigger anger.
Notice the signs of anger.
Go through an anger-reduction routine.
Extract yourself from the situation.
Record how you coped and plan for the future.

At times, hand gestures can be used as cues to the client to stop or alter a negative behavior. For example, a female TBI client had a tendency to touch the person she was next to, straightening a collar, brushing a wrinkle, or removing a stray thread. This behavior, although innocent, could easily be misinterpreted and lead to inappropriate or even aggressive behavior by the other TBI client. With the client's involvement and approval, a discrete hand signal was devised and used to remind her to "stop, think, and act" differently. When the client began reaching out to the person next to her, the therapist would use the signal to cue her to change this behavior.

The twelve steps of Alcoholics Anonymous can be converted to pictures which can greatly benefit the TBI client. Several groups of clients can take part in developing such a set of pictures depicting each step. Therapists can also have each TBI client develop a picture that is meaningful to them. Such visual aids provide clients who have difficulty reading or recognizing words with a picture "worth a thousand words." Also, such client involvement can be critical for acceptance and implementation of such strategies as they are not just given a picture and expected to accept it. The twelve steps of Alcoholics Anonymous can also be converted to twelve steps for head injury (see Exhibit 7.1). When allowed to develop their own behavior, clients' changes are typically more meaningful to them as they "own the product."

Relaxation/Recreation/Adjunctive Therapies

Participation in relaxation therapy is beneficial in teaching arousal reduction techniques for stress management, anger reduction, physical therapy (which may be pain providing), and self-management tech-

EXHIBIT 7.1. The twelve steps for head injury.

1. We acknowledge that our head injury has made our lives difficult and using chemicals may slow down our rehabilitation process.

2. Came to believe that by making responsible decisions for our chemical use we can more rapidly improve.

3. Made a decision to moderate or abstain from chemicals in order to better manage our rehabilitation progress.

4. Made an objective assessment of our past chemical use and its impact on our lives.

5. Admitted to ourselves, our family, and our friends how our chemical use has or would interfere with our rehabilitation.

6. Were entirely ready to make the changes necessary to become more responsible for our chemical use.

7. Willingly asked for help in planning methods to change or stop our chemical use.

8. Made a list of all persons who would support us in making these changes in our chemical use.

9. Made a direct contact with these persons to tell them of the changes we are making and ask for their support and encouragement.

10. Continued to pay attention to our chemical use and to promptly seek assistance if our use increased.

11. Sought through prayer and meditation the strength and determination we need to become the person we know we are.

12. Having been given a second chance at life we commit our thoughts and actions to becoming responsible for ourselves and encouraging our fellow survivors.

Note: While the "Twelve Steps for Head Injury" identified were inspired by the Twelve Steps of Alcoholics Anonymous, they are not really an adaptation. Rather, they were created specifically for this publication, and should not be construed otherwise. AA, which is a program concerned only with recovery from alcoholism, is not in any way affiliated with this publication.

niques. Through the use of planned and guided relaxation, yoga, tai chi, poetry writing, group activities, and community outings, clients can learn new self-management skills and experience sober leisure activities. In addition, nonverbal activities, such as collage making or finger painting, allow clients an opportunity to express themselves to their full ability. For example, in a poetry group, each person can participate, express themselves, and, at times, explore a creative depth unknown and untapped. If a client cannot write, others can assist. If a client has word-finding deficits, peers can learn to patiently wait for the right word to come.

Many TBI clients also experience loneliness, depression, and boredom that can become the triggers for further substance abuse and relapse. Practicing social skills can increase a client's personal sense of attachment to others and social competence. Meeting other people, developing friendships, and experiencing life as a part of a social group increases self-worth. Outings and activities should be selected that lessen the chance for impulse-control problems, and in some cases peers may need to be assigned to assist clients who have eye-hand coordination problems, balance deficits, motor deficits, or endurance problems. Activities or outings that include long walks, crushing masses of people, extraordinary sensory distractors, and unbearable temperatures (such as state fairs) typically result in a less-than-satisfactory experience. Thus, smaller-scale activities such as small county fairs tend to have fewer stimuli and provide a better experience to be enjoyed by all.

Teaching and Utilizing Compensatory Skills

Clients may have had neuropsychological testing performed in the past; however, if not, such testing should be conducted to determine potential strengths and deficits. For example, clients with attention deficits may need preferential seating in group situations. Through observation and questioning the client may be able to report areas of cognitive impairment and behavioral difficulty. When in doubt, ask the client. Clients should be cued to request such accommodation when they find themselves in potentially distracting situations. The therapist should encourage clients to seek out distraction-free environments in which to work or to limit the distractions in the environment. Radios and televisions should not be on when clients are needing to complete other tasks. The therapist should be watchful for signs of fatigue and teach the client to identify their own physical signs and symptoms of fatigue. The therapist should also be looking for withdrawal behaviors in the client, such as signs of confusion and perseveration.

Clients with language-comprehension deficits should be encouraged to use tape recorders, daily planners, notes, or signs as memory aids. The therapist should speak slowly and repeat instructions frequently. When doing a clinical interview, questions should be presented so that a response is required. Stating the question in one- or two-word sentences assists the client in focusing the response and asking for clarification.

If a client has organization-skill deficits, the therapist should teach common routines, for example, support groups should be on the same night each week. Also, tasks should be grouped together; for example, shopping trips for food can include a visit to the pharmacy since many stores have their own in-store pharmacies. Helping clients select a central location for several tasks can decrease confusion.

A PROGRAM FOR TBI PATIENTS
WITH EXECUTIVE DYSFUNCTION

In consideration of the clinical-treatment issues associated with executive dysfunction following brain injury, the following chemical-dependency treatment program is proposed. This treatment program is modeled after the one being used at the Minnesota Neurorehabilitation Hospital (MNH), which is a facility providing comprehensive rehabilitation services to TBI patients with neurobehavioral disorders (Murrey, Helgeson, Courtney, & Starzinski, 1998; Murrey, Starzinski, & LeBlanc, 2003).

Pretreatment Assessment

Prior to beginning treatment it is essential that the therapist ensures that a current and comprehensive neuropsychological evaluation has been completed on the client, which will assess cognitive and executive functioning in addition to the standard CD assessment. The neuropsychological evaluation will provide the CD counselor with an outline of the specific cognitive deficits (memory, attention, and processing) that may be present that could adversely affect the patient's participation in traditional therapies. The neuropsychologist, in conjunction with the CD counselor, also needs to determine (1) any emotional or psychological disturbances directly resulting from the brain injury and (2) the existence and intensity of the anosognosia (lack of awareness of deficit). Table 7.1 provides a set of progressive indicators that can be used in the assessment of anosognosia that is used at

TABLE 7.1. Anosognosia prognostic indicators for persons with traumatic brain injury.

Poorer Prognosis	Better Prognosis
Greater than 2 years postinjury	Less than 1 year postinjury
Global/severe cognitive deficits	Focal/less severe cognitive deficits
Minimal or no acknowledgment of social behavioral deficits	Acknowledgment of social behavioral deficits
High discrepancy between self/other functioning-level reports	Low discrepancy between self/other functioning-level reports
Minimal or no use of compensatory strategies	Use of compensatory strategies
Premorbid behavioral problem history	No premorbid behavioral problem history

the Minnesota Neurorehabilitation Hospital. Clinicians can use this tool by determining which items or indicators on each side of the chart apply to an individual patient. The more items that apply on the "poorer prognosis" side of the chart for the patient suggests (1) a more chronic and severe level of anosognosia and (2) less likelihood of benefitting from traditional CD treatments or insight-oriented treatment alone.

Similar to the model described in Chapter 6 (see Figure 6.1), a four-stage CD treatment model is used at the Minnesota Neurorehabilitation Hospital for TBI patients. These stages are discussed in detail in the next section.

Behavioral and Emotional Stabilization

During the initial phases of treatment, the CD counselor may need to work closely with a neurologist or neuropsychiatrist who can provide necessary pharmacological intervention to reduce levels of agitation, disinhibition, and labile mood. Although some counselors promote a total substance-free recovery model, the use of nonaddictive medications (including antidepressants, antiseizure medications, and atypical neuroleptics) is often essential for TBI patients with executive dyscontrol. Without such interventions the patient may not be able to participate in or benefit from the rehabilitation process.

Psychoeducation, Insight-Building, and Skills-Acquisition Stage

During this phase of intensive CD treatment, intervention needs to include a combination of education on substance abuse and on traumatic brain injury. Imparting this information to the TBI patient must include consideration of his or her cognitive-deficit profile. The use of individualized approaches and strategies to compensate for memory, attention, or processing difficulties may need to be implemented. In this initial stage, the foundation for insight building is laid as the patient is given opportunities to become more aware of his or her behavioral problems in a nonconfrontive and supportive manner. Promoting and gaining compliance by the client is also a primary component of this stage of treatment. In this stage, the treatment team approaches and plans in accordance with clients' deficits and needs. If clients have task-organization deficits, instruct them in the use of a daily planner or a checklist. A client with a foot condition can be given a step-by-step foot-care guide written with his or her involvement so the instruction can contain words meaningful to the client. Cue clients to work in quiet environments and eliminate distractions, and above all cue them to keep their personal items in designated places. Frequently, items of importance are mislaid or lost if placed in drawers—out of sight, out of mind. Some clients need to have considerable open space to organize their personal items, because if the items are in the open and in sight they are not forgotten nor considered lost.

Clients with sequencing deficits should have instructions in as few steps as possible or have information presented one step at a time. Complex tasks with multiple steps should be broken down and numbered. Directions should always be written down. Teaching a client to use a tape recorder or planner can eliminate a great deal of confusion. If problems arise, they should be noted immediately and assistance should be obtained from the therapist. A simple task such as scheduling an appointment with a social worker can be fraught with decisions and choices: When to schedule? How to get there? Does public transportation go there? In such cases, self-cueing strategies are important for success.

Clients with retrieval deficits may have difficulty generalizing new behaviors to the community. The treatment program environment is controlled and predictable, with multiple staff giving the same message in a variety of situations. Cueing is frequent and external assistance is a part of the milieu. The concern arises as to how well these strategies will work when the client is discharged. Having the client use the same visual or auditory cues at home as used in treatment can assist in generalizing the strategy to the community. The client should be discharged with the same memory aid used in treatment, and be reminded to use them to take medications on time, bathe daily, or practice anger control.

Role-playing is also a useful tool to learn new coping skills to avoid risky situations. For example, a young woman had a brother-in-law who would call her and invite her to go out and "party." She had a difficult time saying no. In therapy, another client was assigned to use an office phone to call the first client on the client phone and role-play her brother-in-law asking her to go to a party. As she practiced refusal skills, she became more comfortable at setting limits. The situation mimicked her home environment and she developed a new and critical skill via a simple training technique.

Teaching clients to ask themselves questions when confronted by situations with several possible conclusions can compensate for deficits in problem solving. Using such self-questions as "What else could I do in this situation" or "What would happen if I did that?" is another "stop, think, and act" strategy. Also, teaching clients to scan the environment for cues as to the appropriateness of their behavior, such as facial expressions and other signs of possible social inappropriateness, can cue them to change actions or behavior. For example, a certain client, when the thought of a question would arise, would immediately act on the thought and seek an answer, which often disrupted a group session. He would interrupt the conversation and dominate that conversation until he could resolve his question. His thought process was very linear, and he could focus only on obtaining an answer to his question. He also had difficulty monitoring his own behavior. He was then instructed to ask questions in a single sentence—asking the question, stopping, and waiting for an answer. He was instructed to scan the faces of other clients for signs of disinterest or frustration, and when he would observe these cues from others, he was to "stop talking." Fortunately, this client wanted to be liked, and knew he could become obsessive, so he was motivated to use this technique of practicing scanning others for cues. His effort was recognized and appreciated by his peers and the situation had a mutually agreeable resolution. Although he would still tend to be obsessive, his behaviors improved.

Self-monitoring is a high-level skill and self-questioning can assist with self-monitoring deficits often seen in TBI clients. Helping clients to learn to ask themselves questions such as the following can be very beneficial: Is my speech wandering? Do I understand? Do I need to ask a question? Should I leave this situation? As clients learn to compensate for deficits they can establish more demanding goals and set shorter time lines for completion of tasks. Their ability to compensate also becomes more immediate and spontaneous.

In addition, TBI clients may not initially ask a question if they do not understand. Therapists may ask clients if they understand a particular process or statement, but may only get the standard response: "Sure, I understand." Thus, a critical compensatory skill to teach clients is to ask questions. However, clients need to be positively reinforced for asking questions by the therapist and by peers. While they are developing new skills, the therapist should provide ongoing, nonjudgmental feedback.

Deficits in visual motor skills can be addressed by using written material with large font and clean black characters. In some cases, if using a blackboard, the therapist should print in block format. Clients will need extra time to complete written assignments, and assignments should be short and able to be completed in no more than thirty to forty-five minutes. The client should be able and encouraged to answer in one- or two-word sentences. Groups and tasks should be scheduled at the client's optimal performance time. Usually, morning hours are the most optimal (depending on their reaction to medications).

Skills Proficiency and Generalization Stage

The goal of any change process is to have the new skill accompany the person into the community and his or her personal life. Clients who have generalizing deficits (difficulty transferring new skills into the community) should be given concrete goals and clear, specific tasks. They will also benefit from a predictable schedule and skills in using daily planners and note taking. Role-playing new responses to situations improves recall, and any new behavioral skill should be practiced repeatedly to develop competence. Careful consideration should be given to anticipating situations in which information will be needed, such as on health histories at clinics and job applications. The therapist should assist the client in developing a written document containing such needed information as personal demographics, insurance information, medication list, and health and social service providers (including addresses and telephone numbers). Copies should be kept by the client and another close relative or friend for safekeeping and for future use.

Community Integration Stage

In this stage of therapy, the focus is on integrating the patient back into community support systems depending on the needs and abilities of the client. The beginning of this stage is a reevaluation of the client's abilities to apply and generalize the new skills obtained during the other stages of therapy and determine what level of autonomy and independence would be appropriate in the various community settings. Typically, clients with significant neurobehavioral and executive dysfunction secondary to the brain injury are encouraged to transition to a highly supportive and community-based living or residential program, which may include up to twenty-four-hour-a-day supervision (again depending on the client's level of anosognosia, legal status, and general disability level). However, if the client has developed good insight and has shown significant improvement in managing behaviors and impulses, a less restrictive form of living site may be appropriate. It is suggested, however, that a more cautious approach to the discharge placement be made in light of the very high potential of relapse and difficulties after discharge from such a program. Evaluation for the need for the community-based support and programming in the following areas needs to be considered:

1. *Residential care.* As already mentioned, an evaluation of the client's in-home needs is to be made during this phase of the treatment process to determine the need for in-home supervision and the amount of time during a given day or week that such supervision may be necessary. For this particular type of TBI client, the minimum level of in-home supervision is typically a foster home or semi-independent shared apartment in which a personal care attendant (PCA)

or other professional comes into the home to ensure the client is completing all activities of daily living and taking medications properly.
Such care would also include daily assessments of the client's behavioral status, ensuring that he or she is remaining abstinent from alcohol and other substances. Assessments may also include periodic
urinalyses or blood draws to screen for chemical abuse.

2. *Therapeutic day programs.* The client must also be assessed in
this stage of treatment to determine what level and how much therapeutic programming is needed on a daily or weekly basis. Due to the
significant impulse-control dysfunctions and continued lack of insight (anosognosia) of this type of TBI client, participation in a TBI
and/or CD day treatment program, possibly to include supervised
evening recreational and therapy activities, is not uncommon. However, if the client has been found to be independent or semi-independent in his or her ability to participate in programs and/or employment without supervision and is deemed to be a lower risk for relapse,
then less-structured programming may be needed.

3. *Work programming.* During the community integration assessment, evaluation by the treatment team of the client's abilities during
the work trials to work independently, either in paid employment or
as a volunteer, must be determined. The TBI client's ability to work
may fall along a wide continuum, from inability to participate in any
form of work (including not even being able to participate in a sheltered workshop or extended volunteer position) to being able to participate in competitive employment. However, studies on clients with
significant neurobehavioral disorders secondary to TBI (Murrey et al.,
2003) have shown that only about 50 percent are able to maintain
some form of employment, with less than 10 percent being able to
participate in competitive employment (even with supportive work
coaches and employers). Also, during this stage of the treatment
process, the team must determine what other services would be appropriate for the client once discharged back to the community. Such
services may include individual or group therapy programs with
chemical dependency counselors and/or psychologists. Also, participation in TBI support groups as well as continued follow-up by psychiatry or neurology services need to be determined and recommended. These services, as well as the residential or living situations
and employment or work programming sites need to be developed/

secured before discharge with a complete plan for each area outlined by the treatment team. Ideally, the multidisciplinary treatment team, including the CD therapist, will meet with all caregivers, providers, and employers before the client is discharged from the inpatient program. At this meeting, clear expectations should be made in regard to the client's behaviors with a possible plan for readmission to the inpatient program if the client has a significant relapse or return to preadmission behaviors. Also, it is ideal to have the client visit any residential or day programs and work sites prior to discharge, perhaps including some brief stays/work trials at these locations, having the patient return to the inpatient program for a brief period to review any success or problems during these trials.

CASE EXAMPLE

This case involves a thirty-one-year-old, single male who suffered a TBI from an assault that had occurred six months earlier. He worked as a small-engine mechanic on an as-needed basis and was paid in cash. He had a high school education, but due to illness as a child, missed school for extended periods of time. He had received previous treatment for substance abuse as an outpatient three years earlier. He had been sober for one month after completion of this former treatment. The client did not report mental health problems (past or current). He had been previously diagnosed with kidney disease and received a successful kidney transplant at age twenty-one. He was currently on medications to prevent organ rejection, which were funded through an insurance policy maintained by his parents. He was court referred after receiving a driving under the influence (DUI) citation. There were no other criminal charges or history. His observed behavior was isolative, angry, belligerent, and mistrustful. His mood was noted to be depressed, cautious, and with some observed paranoia. His cognitive deficits included a report of frontal injury with executive dysfunction.

Initial Treatment Assessment: Primary Problems

Treatment resistance: The client was not accepting the need for treatment and did not see alcohol as a problem. He frequented bars to socialize and relax after work.

Recovery environment: The client lived an isolated lifestyle, had few friends, and associated primarily with people who regularly drank. He was living with his parents in their home. He had tried living independently but could not afford to support himself.

Emotional/behavioral/cognitive: The recent injury had left him with little awareness of his deficits (anosognosia) or need for learning compensatory skills. The kidney disease he experienced before the transplant may also have been a contributing factor.

Continued use/relapse potential: He did not have a support network nor a current interest or skills to prevent a relapse. His court involvement and directives called for abstinence and completion of treatment.

Biomedical conditions and complications: He did not believe his chemical use would affect his health or compromise his current transplant status.

Treatment Plan and Approach

The client received individual sessions two times per day to keep him engaged in therapy. He was encouraged to express his dislike of the court system and express his outrage at the recommendation for treatment. The treatment strategy was to roll with the client's resistance and allow him time to incorporate information. The therapist would frequently repeat sobriety and recovery concepts that applied to the client's personal life. The therapist taught the client self-care strategies and would suggest to the client healthier options and offer alternatives for him to consider. The court involvement was never used to confront or coerce the client into accepting recommendations for placement. This was an available tool, but given the client's cautious and mistrustful mood, was not seen as a beneficial approach. The client was also encouraged to fraternize with other clients and participate in recreational outings. He was given the responsibility of assigning unit duties for the other clients, which placed him in a position in which he had to thoughtfully consider the talents and abilities of his peers. An appointment was made with the neuropsychologist, who identified the client's cognitive strengths and deficits.

As treatment progressed, the client became less argumentative and more engaged in the treatment program. From his meeting with the neuropsychologist he gained insight on how identified deficits were affecting his life. He began to recognize how his isolation could be changed, and agreed to move into a supportive living facility for men with cognitive disability and substance-use disorders in a suburb of the city (which provided supervision four hours a day). He recognized his employment was substandard and did not afford him the ability to earn a living. He agreed to accept vocational assistance from the state's Department of Rehabilitative Services. He eventually secured employment in a janitorial position at a local company for which he operated floor-cleaning equipment. A condition of his discharge to the community was his attendance at a biweekly support group.

In summary, cases in which the client has suffered a traumatic brain injury with co-occurring (pre- or postinjury) chemical-dependency issues can be quite complicated and typically require a multidisciplinary approach (with professionals from many different disciplines) and intensive therapeutic programming. As discussed in detail throughout this chapter, assessment and understanding of the client's cognitive and neurobehavioral strengths and weaknesses is essential in the successful development and implementation of the treatment plan and approach for such clients.

APPENDIX: CHEMICAL DEPENDENCY/TRAUMATIC BRAIN INJURY RESOURCES

There are numerous Web sites available for consultation and reference on tapes related to brain injury and/or chemical dependency. The following is a list of such Web sites.

Brain Injury and Disorders

American Brain Tumor Association	www.abta.org
Brain Injury Association	www.biausa.org
Depression and Related Affective Disorders Association	www.drada.org
The Epilepsy Foundation	www.efa.org
Learning Disabilities Association of America	www.ldanatl.org
The National Institute of Mental Health	www.nimh.nih.gov
National Spinal Cord Injury Association	www.spinalcord.org
National Stroke Association	www.stroke.org

Chemical Dependency

Alcoholics Anonymous	www.alcoholics-anonymous.org
Online Intergroup of Alcoholics Anonymous	www.aa-intergroup.org
Recovery.org—various resources	www.recovery.org
Sober 24—live meetings and chat room	www.sober24.com
Women for Sobriety	www.womenforsobriety.org

Many states have their own associations, and the national organization may have links to these state organizations. Each organization's home page will have links to other sites that can be examined in each area of interest. Computers are available at public libraries and other public venues in which those without home computers can access these sites. In many communities there are resources that assist people who need computers with funds to purchase this equipment. Frequently, there is low or no cost associated with the acquisition for persons with disabilities. In addition, voice-recognition software allows individuals with motor deficits the opportunity to communicate.

The Brain Injury Association of America's Web site offers links to the following topics, available at <www.biausa.org/Pages/links_resources.html>:

Case management	Military
Chat rooms	Other organizations
Education	Personal pages
Employment	Prevention
General information	Professional/rehab
International associations	Software/computing
International languages	Surveys
Kids and parents	TBI-related organizations
Legal profession	Technical
Legislation	

BIBLIOGRAPHY

Arenth, P.M., Bogner, J.A., Corrigan, J.D., & Schmidt, L. (2001). The Utility of the Substance Abuse Subtle Screening Inventory for Use with Individuals with Brain Injury. *Brain Injury, 15*(6): 499-510.

Bogner, J.A., Corrigan, J.D., et al. (1997). Integrating Substance Abuse Treatment and Vocational Rehabilitation Following Traumatic Brain Injury. *Journal of Head Trauma Rehabilitation, 12*(5): 57-71.

Corrigan, J.D. (1995). Substance Abuse As a Mediating Factor in Outcome from Traumatic Brain Injury. *Archives of Physical Medicine and Rehabilitation, 76*(4): 302-309.

Corrigan, J.D., Bogner, J.A., et al. (1999). Substance Abuse and Brain Injury. In M. Rosenthal, E.R. Griffith, J.D. Miller, and J. Kreutzer (Eds.), *Rehabilitation of the Adult and Child with Traumatic Brain Injury, Third Edition*. Philadelphia: F.A. Davis Co.

DeFord, M.S. (2002). Repeated Mild Brain Injury. *Myths and New Directions Brain Injury Source, 6*(1): 32-37.

Delmonico, R.L., Hanley-Peterson, P., & Englander, J. (1998). Group Psychotherapy for Persons with Traumatic Brain Injury: Management of Frustration and Substance Abuse. *The Journal of Head Trauma Rehabilitation, 13*(6): 10-22.

Goldstein, R.C., & Levin, H.S. (1995). Neurobehavioral Outcome of Traumatic Brain Injury: Coma, the Vegetative State, and the Minimally Responsive State. *The Journal of Head Trauma Rehabilitation, 10*(1): 57-73.

Grace, J., Stout, J.C., & Malloy, P.F. (1999). Assessing Frontal Lobe Behavioral Syndromes with the Frontal Lobe Personality Scale. *Psychological Assessment Resources, 6*(3): 269-284.

Karol, R.L. (2003). *Neuropsychosocial Intervention: The Practical Treatment of Severe Behavioral Dyscontrol After Acquired Brain Injury.* Boca Raton, FL: CRC.

Karol, R. & Sparedeo, F. (1991). *Alcohol, Drugs and Brain Injury.* Lynn, MA: New Medico Head Injury System.

Kramer, T.R., & Hoisington, D. (1992). Use of AA and NA in the Treatment of Chemical Dependencies of Traumatic Brain Injury Survivors. *Brain Injury, 6*(1): 81-88.

Kreutzer, J.S., Witol, A.D., et al. (1996). A Prospective Longitudinal Multicenter Analysis of Alcohol Use Patterns Among Persons with Traumatic Brain Injury. *Journal of Head Trauma Rehabilitation, 11*(5): 58-78.

Lezak, M.D. (1993). Newer Contributions to the Neuropsychological Assessment of Executive Functions. *The Journal of Trauma Rehabilitation, 8*(1): 24-31.

Miller, W.R. (1999). Enhancing Motivation for Change in Substance Abuse Treatment. #35 Treatment Improvement Protocol Series, Substance Abuse and Mental Health Services Administration. Rockville, MD: Department of Health and Human Services.

Moore, D. (1998). Substance Use Disorder Treatment for People with Physical and Cognitive Disabilities. #29 Treatment Improvement Protocol Series, Substance Abuse and Mental Health Services Administration. Rockville, MD: Department of Health and Human Services.

Murrey, G.J., Helgeson, S., Courtney, C., & Starzinski, D. (1998). State Coordinated Services for Traumatic Brain Injury Survivors: Toward a Model Delivery System. *Journal of Head Trauma Rehabilitation, 13*(6): 72-81.

Murrey, G.J., Starzinski, D., & LeBlanc, A. (2003). Patient Neurobehavioral Rehabilitation Program for Persons with Traumatic Brain Injury: Overview and Outcome Data for the Minnesota Neurorehabilitation Hospital. *Brain Injury.*

Murrey, G.J., Starzinski, D.T., and LeBlanc, A.J. (2004). Base Rates of Traumatic Brain Injury History in Adults Admitted to State Psychiatric Hospitals: A 3-Year Study. *Rehabilitation Psychology, 49*(3): 259-261.

Prigatano, G.P. (1999). *Principles of Neuropsychological Rehabilitation.* New York: Oxford University Press.

Sohlberg, M.M., Matteer, C.A., & Struss, D.T. (1993). Contemporary Approaches to the Management of Executive Control Dysfunction. *The Journal of Head Trauma Rehabilitation, 8*(1): 45-58.

Strand, L. (2002). *Learners with Disabilities, Adult Basic Education Resource Guide*. Resource manual funded under a 2001-2002 ABE Statewide Supplemental Services Grant. New Hope, MN: Dzine Publications.

Strauss, D.L. (2002). *Moving Forward: Issues and Insights*. Selected presentations from the Mayo Brain Injury Conference, Rochester, MN: 79-86.

Trudel, T.M., Tyron, W.W., & Purdum, C.M. (1998). Awareness of Disability and Long-Term Outcome After Traumatic Brain Injury. *Rehabilitation Psychology*, *43*(4): 267-281.

Chapter 8

All-Digital, Real-Time EEG Feedback with Open and Closed Head Trauma

Margaret E. Ayers

INTRODUCTION AND OVERVIEW

Traumatic brain injury is an important public health problem. In a 2004 report, the Centers for Disease Control and Prevention reported that at least 1.4 million people sustain a traumatic brain injury in the United States each year. Of those, about 50,000 die, 235,000 are hospitalized, and 1.1 million are treated and released from emergency rooms (Langlois, Rutland-Brown, and Thomas, 2004). However, many seek medical care that does not involve emergency room conditions. Brain injury is not considered a disease, yet it can affect functioning in many ways. Symptoms may include difficulty with learning, cognition, memory, vision, sensitivity to light and sound, headaches, immunity, dizziness and mood swings, reversal of words, problems with judgment, appropriate behavior and speech.

Biofeedback is a noninvasive process of furnishing information about various body functions through sound, vision, or sensation. Through such feedback a person can gain voluntary control over the specific physiological function that is being sampled. For example, a digital thermometer can be placed on the finger of someone with tension headaches to measure hand temperature, which is displayed in digital numbers. Learning to relax the body raises the digital thermometer reading and, as a result, reduces the tension headaches. Historically, electrical activity of the muscle has been recorded by electromyographic feedback and displayed on a video screen in front of the client, usually along with an audible signal that increases in volume as the muscle activity increases. According to Ayers (1981), individuals with no feeling in their fingers and arm after having strokes could learn to increase hand opening with muscle feedback.

Electroencephalograph (EEG) biofeedback measures brain waves to help reduce brain-injury sequelae and improve neurological and behavioral functions. Brain-wave feedback was first performed by Joseph Kamiya in 1967, during which subjects were required to guess whether they were producing alpha waves whenever given a signal (Kamiya, 1967). During these studies, subjects improved significantly in identifying alpha-wave production, some as much as 50 percent on the first day of training. The first subject correctly identified alpha-wave production 65 percent of the time on day two, and 85 percent of the time on day three. In subsequent research conducted by Barbara Brown (1970), the researcher was able to train subjects to produce alpha waves on demand. Both controlled and noncontrolled research studies in brain-wave biofeedback have since been published on patients with migraines, stress-related disorders, head trauma, cerebral palsy, stroke, ADD and ADHD, Parkinson's disease, coma, epilepsy, and learning disabilities (see Byers, 1998). Thus, patients with a variety of medical conditions have benefited from the clinical application of EEG biofeedback training.

EEG BIOFEEDBACK
WITH BRAIN-INJURED CLIENTS

Persons with brain injury often present with a multitude of physical, cognitive, and emotional problems. According to Rizzo and Tranel (1996), the symptoms of brain trauma may include impairments in concentration and attention, and may cause headache and neck discomfort; dizziness or vertigo; mood changes such as depression, insomnia, apathy, fatigue, blurred vision, and anhedonia (loss of interest in pleasurable activities). In addition, Ayers (2002) and Quattrocchi and colleagues (1992) reported that people with brain injury are at a high risk for sickness and for developing chronic immune-system problems (since the brain is the regulator of the immune system). For many years, nonpenetrating, closed brain injury has been considered a mild head injury. Recently, however, researchers have found that the term *mild brain injury* may be an oxymoron.

Bergsneider and colleagues (2000) studied positron-emission tomography (PET) scans that showed the glucose levels in brain cells. Examining the PET scans of forty-two patients with mild to severe concussions within thirty days postinjury showed that glucose metabolism was just as low in mild TBI patients as it was in the severely brain-injured patients. In this study, researchers considered a glucose metabolism of 4.9mg/100g per minute below normal, and found the mean glucose level for all of the patients was 3.9mg/100g per minute with a variability of plus or minus 0.6. In the future, PET scans may be valuable diagnostic tools to be used in addition to neuropsychological tests and EEG.

The recording of brain-wave activity utilizing the EEG has evolved from its analog ink pen invention by Hans Berger in 1929, to digital machines used for evoked potentials, to all-digital, real-time recording. Duffy (1986) invented quantitative analysis of the digital EEG (QEEG). The quantitative analysis of the EEG used the mathematical fast Fourier transform (FFT) spectrum with results expressed as the square root of the spectral power. Samples of up to 128 per minute were then added and averaged. Individuals such as Gevins and colleagues (1994), Wong (1991), Thatcher and colleagues (1989), and Soherg and Ebersole (1993) studied and applied averaged or derived secondary data. With the FFT EEG, clinicians no longer see the raw primary EEG that was used with the analog pen-and-ink EEG. The pen-and-ink EEG could not move fast enough to pick up details of EEG patterns and, as a result, individuals with major brain dysfunction often had normal analog pen-and-ink EEGs. Therefore, people with brain injury may present with normal EEGs. Since magnetic resonance imaging (MRI) and computerized tomography (CT) scans show only tumors or lesions, such as in a stroke, patients with brain injury may also have normal MRI and CT scans.

However, the FFT secondary QEEG gives different data from that of primary analog or all-digital, real-time EEG feedback systems. Research and clinical neurofeedback based on averaging EEG data often gives erroneous information to clients and clinicians. Once research data are averaged in a power spectrum, the original primary EEG cannot be displayed. In addition, frequency values averaged in a power spectrum are real, mathematically speaking, but may not exist in the real EEG. However, the squared FFT wave represents a finite number of sine waves that do not appear in the original EEG. Also, FFT low frequencies appearing in power-spectral analyses have increased power because of the mathematical logarithm. When using a Fourier system, closed brain injury clients present with high power in delta (0 to 4 Hz) wave when no delta exist in the original primary EEG. In addition, the FFT delta frequency may be artificial or consist of complex wave forms that cause delta waves to appear when they do not exist in the raw EEG. Even in analog EEG, the complex wave forms or spikes appear in the 4 to 7 Hz range, which appear as delta waves in the FFT EEG. Thus, only real-time, all-digital EEG can display the complete complex EEG patterns that cannot be seen in averaged, derived, or analog measures.

Even though Thatcher and colleagues (1989) created an FFT-averaged secondary QEEG base for brain trauma, many individuals with TBI would show normal QEEGs. In addition, QEEGs do not detect individuals with postviral infections or chemical poisoning but instead classify them as head injured. Therefore, the primary EEG pattern must be reviewed to determine if a brain injury pattern is present. As a result, individuals with TBI are often erroneously accused of malingering or are labeled as having post-traumatic stress disorder. However, Ayers and Heyser (1983) discovered that persons with brain injury show a specific EEG pattern that is clearly different from that of malingerers. The EEG pattern consists of phasic single spikes attached to theta or 4 to 7 Hz activity. An obvious conclusion is that once brain injury EEG patterns are identified, individuals might be able to learn to inhibit the behaviors detected in the abnormal EEG by utilizing the EEG feedback.

Ayers (1987, 1993; Ayers and Heyser, 1983) was the first to have subjects try to inhibit the brain trauma EEG pattern of phasic single spikes at 4 to 7 Hz activity. In 1987, Ayers successfully had 250 subjects inhibit 4 to 7 Hz and produce 15 to 18 Hz on both T4C4 right sensorimotor cortex and T3C3 left sensorimotor cortex (based on the International 10-20 System of Electrode Placement). The activity was measured for fifteen minutes on each side for a total of twenty-four sessions. An EEG was taken after each set of six sessions for a total of four EEGs. Symptomatology was recorded for each client, and none were taking sedatives. Individuals were asked to report any changes in symptomology in each session. The purpose was to determine whether any consistent pattern of symptomology change existed.

Following EEG neurofeedback, individuals reported an increase in energy and a decrease in depression and temper outbursts after the first six sessions. Throughout the next six sessions individuals reported a decrease in sensitivity to sound and light and an increased attention span. In the subsequent six sessions all individuals had a reduction in reported dizziness. The headaches that were clinically considered to be vascular in nature seemed to disappear in the final six sessions. Subjects also reported increased libido and less reversal of letters or words. In the twenty-four feedback sessions, only fifteen of the 250 subjects reported significant improvement in short-term memory. Subsequent research (Ayers, 1987) suggests that it may take up to forty sessions to show significant improvement in return of short-term memory for TBI clients. In addition, after six sessions, most phasic spikes shown on the EEG decreased. In the following six sessions, all spikes were gone, but slow 4 to 7 Hz activity remained. In the next six sessions, 4 to 7 Hz activity did decrease. In the last six sessions, most 4 to 7 Hz activity was totally eliminated. The primary implication of this study was that the brain has a developmental hierarchy of motor control; the "simplest" deficits seem to disappear first (e.g., all subjects reported an increase in energy) and the more complex brain tasks (e.g., short-term memory) tend to improve/return last.

Ayers's (1993) controlled study compared EEG biofeedback treatment of right hemispheric brain-injured individuals suffering from anxiety or panic attacks with traditional psychotherapy treatment. The group treated with EEG biofeedback were trained to inhibit the abnormal phasic spike and 4 to 7 Hz activity with feedback totally eliminated their anxiety and panic attacks. However, the group receiving only clinical psychotherapy showed a reduction of their anxiety symptoms but still presented with panic attacks. One conclusion that might be drawn from these studies is that many tools ranging from clinical psychotherapy to ice packs might help with symptom relief, but unless one goes directly to the brain (our human engine), symptoms may not go away. Ignoring the brain is akin to one taking a car into the auto mechanic and saying "check the tires, ignition, muffler, battery, and generator, but whatever you do, don't check the engine." The mechanic might think that you were having a brain lapse. By treating the brain directly, permanent changes can be made to defective brain trauma patterns. What then happens is that the EEG normalizes and the original unique EEG pattern of that individual is restored to a healthy state.

In further research, Hoffman (1995) reported success with using EEG feedback with QEEG to map traumatic brain injury. Hoffman demonstrated successful inhibition of theta-wave activity and simultaneously produced beta wave in brain-injured clients while also improving their symptomology. Open head injury clients may have more severe symptomology because of skull penetration. Corville (1958) discovered that the temporal lobes often are damaged during impact by the bony middle fossa of the skull, causing lesions or brain trauma resulting in psychomotor epilepsy. As a result, intermittent delta activity of 3 to 4 Hz is often observed in open head trauma for which a lesion can be documented on a CT scan or MRI. The delta and theta will both be higher in amplitude in both open and closed head trauma at the site of impact. However, sharp waves (over seventy milliseconds wide at the bottom) are usually seen only in severe open head trauma or stroke; theta and beta amplitudes are elevated in both open and closed head trauma, but are highest in open head trauma. Symptomology in open head trauma also tends to be more profound than in closed head trauma. Sometimes in closed head trauma a CNS depression with overall lowered microvoltage amplitudes will be seen on the EEG. It is thus apparent that individual beta amplitude increases are an attempt to compensate for CNS depression by overriding the excessive theta or delta.

For treatment of stroke patients, neurological site-specific EEG feedback in the sensorimotor cortex (the area that controls leg movement and sensation) is necessary. The International 10-20 System of Electrode Placement just behind Fz (mid-frontal) and in front of Pz (mid-parietal) is made. In cases in which a posttrauma speech disorder is present, feedback should be done directly on Wernicke's and Broca's speech areas of the brain (or F7T5 in the 10-20 system). Neurological site-specific EEG feedback often immediately improves ambulation of the leg area and it also leads to improvement in speech based on Wernicke's and Broca's speech centers.

Ayers (2002) observed that in open head trauma (more than in closed head trauma) immune problems are quite prevalent. Clients will report more colds, general malaise, and increased fatigue. Severe open head trauma may result in suppression of cellular immunity according to Quattrocchi and colleagues (1992). Also, according to Quattrocchi and colleagues (1991), helper T-cell function and lymphokine-activated killer cell cytotoxicity is impaired. However, after inhibiting the theta and phasic EEG spikes at the site of the injury, clients will report less illness and fatigue, and an improved sense of well-being. Open head trauma also often results in increased temper, mood swings, poor social skills, impulsive sexual behavior, poor judgment, balance problems, and neuroanatomical site-specific deficits.

The reality of brain plasticity in brain trauma patients is one of the first profound implications of all-digital, real-time EEG feedback. It was Erickson and colleagues (1998) who discovered that the human hippocampus (in the subcortex region of the brain) retains the ability to generate neurons throughout life. It was previously thought that the brain did not grow new cells. However, Lowenstein and Parent (1999) observed that growing of new brain cells, or neurogenesis, can also have negative effects, resulting in such symptoms as prolonged seizures that can cause increased neurogenesis in the dentate gyrus after brain injury. Toxins also can cause increased glia scaring or abnormal neurogenesis. Thus, the brain injury is far from being cured. Since the hippocampus is the main generator of theta waves, it is possible that excessive neurogenesis of hippocampal cells could be restrained by inhibiting excessive theta activity. Using all-digital, real-time EEG feedback treatment at 250,000 samples per second (not averaged), with less than a 1,000-second delay between brainwave production, can help patients learn to inhibit sharp waves, phasic spikes, and 4 to 7 Hz theta waves and thus take advantage of brain plasticity. This therapeutic method thus allows the central nervous system to "unconsciously" receive feedback like touch, hearing, and eyesight about the brain and to immediately self-correct the impaired system. It is similar to looking in a mirror to comb your hair the way that you want it to appear. The computer screen with the brain waves in all-digital, real-time feedback is the mirror to "comb" or adjust brain waves into place.

TREATMENT CASES

Figures 8.1 and 8.2 are of an EEG of a closed head brain injury client who had suffered a TBI after a motorcycle accident. Note the pretreatment phasic spikes and 4 to 7 Hz activity prior to inhibition of theta (see Figure 8.1). The theta prior to all-digital, real-time EEG feedback was 2.22 microvolts, which was decreased to 1.57 after feedback treatment (see Figure 8.2).

Figures 8.3 and 8.4 show pre- and postbiofeedback treatment EEGs of a child who was hit by a car and suffered an open head trauma at the age of eight. He did not receive biofeedback treatment until age seventeen. He was in a wheelchair, could not walk, his speech was barely intelligible, he had extreme spasticity, and had a shortened arm and leg on the right side from a posttrauma stroke. The patient's pretreatment EEG is shown in Figure 8.3. After fifty feedback sessions, he was walking without assistance, speaking slowly but clearly, and functioning independently. On the left side, where his stroke occurred from the open head trauma (T3C3 sensorimotor cortex), the theta was 4.25 microvolts of theta, and following all-digital, real-time EEG feedback, the theta was 2.10 microvolts (see Figure 8.4).

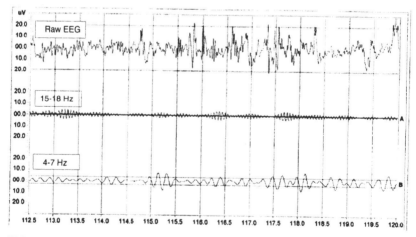

FIGURE 8.1. Case 1—Pretreatment EEG. This individual had a closed head injury on the right side due to a motorcycle crash. The signature is characterized by the pattern of phasic single spikes and excessive 4 to 7 Hz activity. His symptoms included loss of short-term memory, inappropriate social judgment, aggression, mood swings, poor concentration, and sensitivity to sound and light.

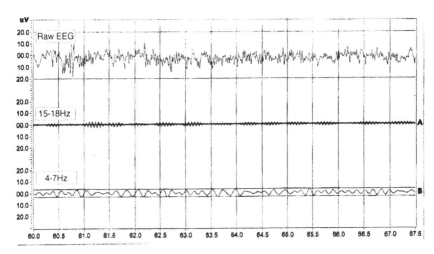

FIGURE 8.2. Case 1—Posttreatment EEG. This is session eighteen in which this individual trained himself to inhibit spikes and excessive 4 to 7 Hz activity. Short-term memory returned, social judgment became more appropriate, mood improved, concentration improved, and he became less sensitive to sound and light.

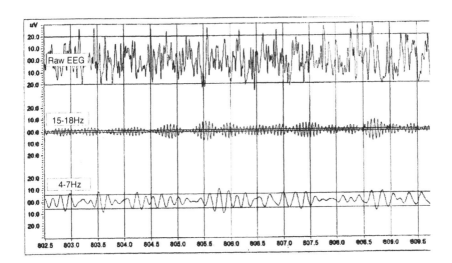

FIGURE 8.3. Case 2—Pretreatment EEG. Seventeen-year-old with open head injury due to having been hit by a car at the age of eight. Theta is 4.25 microvolts. He is in a wheelchair, cannot walk, and is barely understandable. He has extreme spasticity from a stroke on the right side.

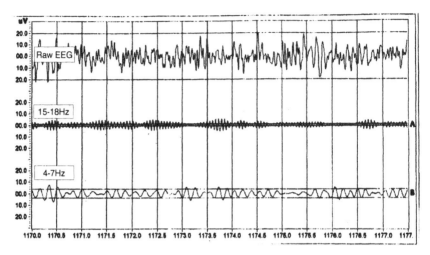

FIGURE 8.4. Case 2—Posttreatment EEG. Boy who was injured at the age of eight and received feedback at the age of seventeen. After feedback theta is 2.10 microvolts.

CONCLUSION

Any health professional, such as a psychologist, physician, osteopath, chiropractor, acupuncturist, nurse, speech therapist, or occupational therapist, can receive specialized training in biofeedback therapy. Education in brain function benefits all professionals working with patients with head trauma.

APPENDIX: ADDITIONAL RESOURCES

Ayers, M.E. (1969). Therapeutic intervention with an adolescent drug abuse population. *Washington Guidance Journal, 9,* 15.

Ayers, M.E. (1971). *Conflict intervention with drug abuse.* Paper presented at Washington State Personnel and Guidance Association Convention on Conflict Intervention. Ocean Shores, Washington.

Ayers, M.E. (1982). *Landmarks in primary unipolar depression.* Paper presented at Intra-Research Science Foundation, University of Southern California, Los Angeles, California.

Ayers, M.E. (1983). Electroencephalographic feedback and head trauma. In Heyser, G. (Ed.), *Head and Neck Trauma: The Latest Information and Perspec-*

tives on Patients with a Less-Than-Optimal Recovery (pp. 244-257). UCLA Neuropsychiatric Institute.

Ayers, M.E. (1985). *EEG neurofeedback for depression and hyperactivity.* Paper presented at the CANCH-ACLD State Conference. Orange, California.

Ayers, M.E. (1985). *EEG neurofeedback brain research with stroke, head injury and epilepsy.* Paper presented at the California Association of Post-Secondary Educators of the Disabled State Conference. Sacramento, California.

Ayers, M.E. (1985). Healing and the brain. *Epilepsy Support Program Newsletter,* 13(1), 8-9.

Ayers, M.E. (1985). *Left hemisphere head trauma learning disabilities and electroencephalography training to correct resulting learning dysfunction.* Paper presented at the International ACLD Conference. Costa Mesa, California.

Ayers, M.E. (1987, December). Electroencephalographic neurofeedback and closed head injury of 250 individuals. *National Head Injury Syllabus, Head Injury Frontiers,* 380.

Ayers, M.E. (1988). Long term clinical treatment follow-up of EEG neurofeedback for epilepsy. *Epilepsy Support Program Newsletter,* 3(2), 8-9.

Ayers, M.E. (1990). *All children learn differently.* A videotape published by Learning Disabilities Association of California, Orange County. Santa Ana, California.

Ayers, M.E. (1991). *A controlled study of EEG neurofeedback training and clinical psychotherapy for right hemispheric closed head injury.* Paper presented at the National Head Injury Foundation Conference. Los Angeles, California.

Ayers, M.E. (2001). Response to the question, "Have you seen any negative effects associated with EEG neurofeedback?" *Journal of Neurotherapy,* 4(4), 63-65.

Ayers, M.E. (1999). Assessing and treating open head trauma, coma, and stroke using real-time digital EEG neurofeedback. In J. Evans (Ed.), *Quantitative EEG and Neurofeedback* (pp. 203-222). San Diego: Academic Press.

Bhat, J., Chee, E., Lurie, Y., Bhat, N., and Ayers, M. (2001). Neurofeedback to treat insomnia in congestive heart failure patients: An innovative approach. Abstract. *Applied Psychophysiology and Biofeedback,* 26(3), 245.

Sterman, M.B., Ayers, M.E., and Goodman, S.J. (1976). Effects of SMR suppression on EEG and motor patterns in quadriplegic patient. *Biofeedback and Self-Regulation,* 1(3), 340-341.

Taylor, P., Ayers, M.E., and Tom, G.F. (1981). *Electromyometric, biofeedback therapy: A report on a study of the utilization of electroencephalography (Neuroanalyzer) for the treatment of cerebral vascular lesion syndromes.* Biofeedback and Advanced Therapy Institute, Inc., Los Angeles, California.

REFERENCES

Ayers, M.E. (1981). A report on a study of the utilization of electroencephalography for the treatment of cerebral vascular lesion syndromes. In Taylor, L., Ayers,

M.E., and Tom, C. (Eds.), *Electromyometric Biofeedback Therapy* (pp. 244-257). Los Angeles, CA: Biofeedback and Advanced Therapy Institute.

Ayers, M.E. (1987, December). Electroencephalographic neurofeedback and closed head injury of 250 individuals. *National Head Injury Syllabus, Head Injury Frontiers*, 380.

Ayers, M.E. (1991). Electroencephalographic neurofeedback apparatus and method for bioelectric frequency inhibition and facilitation. *Official Gazette*, U.S. Patent Office, Patent Number 5,024,235, June 18.

Ayers, M.E. (1993). A controlled study of EEG neurofeedback training and clinical psychotherapy for right hemispheric closed head injury. *Biofeedback and Self-Regulation*, 18(3), 148.

Ayers, M.E. (2002). *Brain immunity using all digital real time EEG feedback.* Paper presented at the American College for Advancement (ACAM) Fall Conference, Phoenix, Arizona, November.

Ayers, M. and Heyser, G. (Ed.) (1983). Department of Continuing Education in Health Sciences. UCLA School of Medicine, Los Angeles: Electroencephalographic feedback and head trauma. In *Head and Neck Trauma: The Latest Information and Perspectives on Patients with Less Than Optimal Recovery*, 8-11.

Bergsneider, M., Hovda, D.A., Lee, S.M., Kelly, D.F., McArthur, D.L., Vespa, P.M., Lee, J.H., Huang, S.-C., Martin, N.A., Phelps, M.E., and Becker, D.P. (2000). Dissociation of cerebral glucose metabolism and level of consciousness during the period of metabolic depression following human traumatic brain injury. *Journal of Neurotrauma*, 5(17), 389.

Brown, B. (1970). Recognition of aspects of consciousness thought association with EEG alpha rhythm. *Psychophysiology*, 6, 442.

Byers, A. (1998). *Byers Neurotherapy Reference Library* (2nd edition). Wheat Ridge, CO: The Association for Applied Psychophysiology and Biofeedback.

Corville, C.B. (1958). Traumatic lesions of the temporal lobe as the essential cause of psychomotor epilepsy. In Baldwin, M. and Bailey, E. (Eds.), *Temporal Lobe Epilepsy* (pp. 220-239). Springfield, IL: Thomas.

Duffy, F.H. (1986). *Topographic Mapping of Brain Electrical Activity.* Boston, MA: Butterworth.

Erickson, P.S., PerFilieva, E., Biork-Eriksson, T., Alborn, A.M., Nordborg, C., Peterson, D.A., and Gage, F.H. (1998). Neurogenesis in the adult human hippocampus. *Nature Medicine*, 4(11), 1313-1317.

Gevins, A., Martin, H., Bryckett, P., Desmond, J., and Reuters, B. (1994). High resolution EEG: 124 channel recording spatial reblurring and MRI integration. *EEG Clinical Neurophysiological*, 90, 337-358.

Hoffman, D. (1995). Diagnosis and treatment of head injury. *Journal of Neurotherapy*, 1(1), 14-21.

Kamiya, J. (1967). Conscious control of brain waves. *Psychology Today*, 1, 57.

Langlois, J.A., Rutland-Brown, W., and Thomas, K.E. (2004). *Traumatic Brain Injury in the United States: Emergency Department Visits, Hospitalizations, and Deaths.* Atlanta (GA): Centers for Disease Control and Prevention, National Center for Injury Prevention and Control. Retrieved August 14, 2005, from CDC Web site.

Lowenstein, D.H., and Parent, J.M. (1999). Brain, heal thyself. *Science,* 283(19), 1126-1127.

Quattrocchi, K., Frank, E., Miller, C., Amin, A., Issel, B., and Wagner, F. (1991). Impairment of helper T-cell function and lymphokine-lymphokine-activated killer cytotoxicity following severe head injury. *Journal of Neurosurgery,* 75, 766-773.

Quattrocchi, K., Miller, C., Wagner, F., DeNardy, S., Quodov, K., and Franke, F. (1992). Cell mediated immunity in severely head injured patients: The role of suppressor lymphocytes and serum factors. *Journal of Neurosurgery,* 77(5), 694-699.

Rizzo, M. and Tranel, D. (1996). Overview of head injury and post concussive syndrome. In Rizzo, M. and Tranel, D. (Eds.), *Head Injury and Postconcussive Syndrome* (pp. 1-18). Philadelphia: Elsevier.

Soherg, M., and Ebersole, J.S. (1993). Models of brain sources. *Brain Topography,* 5(4), 419-423.

Thatcher, R.W., Walker, R.S., and Gerson, I. (1989). EEG discriminate analysis of mild head trauma. *EEG Clinical Neurophysiology,* 73, 94-106.

Wong, P.K.H. (1991). Source modeling of the rolandic focus. *Brain Topography,* 4(2), 105-112.

Chapter 9

Craniosacral Therapy
for Traumatic Brain Injury Clients
with Neurobehavioral Disorders

Ann Wedel

INTRODUCTION AND OVERVIEW

Craniosacral therapy is a gentle, nonintrusive, hands-on healing technique utilized by experienced therapists to help the physical body release restricted tissues and restore optimal physical, emotional, behavioral, and cognitive functions (Burget, 2002). It is an alternative medicine technique that is readily able to work with and enhance the effects of traditional allopathic treatments. It can be a very effective means of helping people work through and release chronic pain. Basically, it is a transformational manual therapy technique used to help people suffering from orthopedic and neurological problems to function at a higher level (Reuben, 1987; Smoley, 1991; Upledger, 1996).

The name *craniosacral* refers to a semienclosed membrane system named after the bones involved in the anchoring of this system: the cranium and the sacrum (Burke, 1997). Even though the name implies anatomic structures involving the head and the pelvis, this can be misleading. Craniosacral therapy can be used as a healing tool throughout the body to assist in rejuvenating scarred or restricted structures such as the brain, the bones, the muscles, the nerves, the vessels, and the organs.

The craniosacral system is composed of the bones of the skull, face, and mouth, which make up the cranium, sacrum, cerebrospinal fluid, brain, spinal cord, and connective tissues. The formation of the craniosacral system starts embryologically and remains functional throughout one's life, even slightly past death (Upledger and Vredevoogd, 1983). It has been found to be the last physiological rhythm to stop following death and is present in all vertebrates. Craniosacral therapy can help restore both physical and emotional stability in one's life. To understand craniosacral therapy, it is important to understand that the craniosacral system is a semienclosed hydraulic system (Heinrich, 1991b). The craniosacral system produces a slight but very significant hydraulic pressure that is transmitted throughout the system. This pressure originates in the choroid plexuses in the first and third ventricles of the brain. The choroid plexuses create cerebrospinal fluid by filtering fluid out of the blood. Since the craniosacral system is a semienclosed system it creates a hydraulic pressure that builds as the amount of cerebrospinal fluid increases, thereby bathing the brain and spinal cord throughout the entire dura mater. When the fluid moves, the membranes or dural tube in which these membranes reside also move. The resulting slight motion caused from the increase and decrease in hydraulic pressure can be felt throughout the entire body. The most common areas in which these pressures are felt are on the head, sacrum, and coccyx because these areas attach directly into the membranes of the craniosacral system that enclose the cerebrospinal fluid (Smoley, 1991).

An internal physiological regulating mechanism within the cranium creates the rate of the craniosacral rhythm. This neuromechanism involves the stretch and compression receptors in the sagittal suture (Retzlaff et al., 1978; Retzlaff et al., 1976; Retzlaff et al., 1979; Reuben, 1987). As cerebrospinal fluid is manufactured and released in the choroid plexuses, a stretch response in the sagittal sutures occurs. This response then gives a signal to the choroid plexuses in the lateral and the third ventricles of the brain to briefly halt or reduce production of the cerebrospinal fluid. This change in cerebrospinal fluid production results in stopping or significantly reducing the inflow of fluid into the dura. As the production of cerebrospinal fluid is reduced or stopped, the sagittal suture compresses one parietal bone against the other, creating a nerve signal to the choroid plexuses in the ventricular system of the brain, which causes cerebral spinal fluid production to begin again (Reuben, 1987).

This cerebrospinal fluid production occurs for about three seconds and then is shut down for about three seconds, which gives the system its rhythmical rise and fall of pressure (thus its subtle movement). It is this movement or rhythm that is so important to craniosacral therapists and craniosacral treatments (Smoley, 1991; Cohen, 1989a,b,c). The arachnoid villae, which are located in many areas within the dural tube, reabsorb cerebrospinal fluid back into the venous system. The villae are most concentrated in the sagittal venus sinus. The entire craniosacral mechanism must work harmoniously to create this rhythm, and any tension in the membrane system can have a disruptive effect upon cerebrospinal fluid production and ultimately on health and vitality (Upledger and Vredevoogd, 1983).

The dural membrane is the internal connective tissue lining of the bone structure of the skull. It attaches to the inner lining of all the cranial bones. As the dural membrane extends down the spinal canal it becomes the dural tube. This tube attaches to the foramen magnum of the occiput, to the second and third cervical vertebrae, and to the back of the second sacral segment. It exits the vertebral canal and blends into the sacrococcygeal complex. It is for this reason that the sacrum will move in rhythm with the cranium (Upledger and Vredevoogd, 1983).

Among the more subtle physiological body movements to palpate is the rhythmical internal and external rotation of the total body through the fascia, which is a normal response to the craniosacral rhythm. A good craniosacral therapist is able to assess this rhythm via the proprioceptive senses (Smoley, 1991). With hands placed gently on the patient's head, this craniosacral rhythm/movement can be felt as a slight widening or expansion of the head (flexion phase), a pause, a slight contraction or narrowing or elongation of the head (extension phase), then another pause; this rhythm repeats over and over again. With hands placed on the body during the flexion phase, the therapist detects the entire body slightly externally rotate or widen. In the extension phase, the entire body will slightly internally rotate. Similar to the feeling on the head, there is a slight neutral phase between flexion and extension during which the body rests or pauses momentarily. Any lack of symmetry in the rhythmical motion throughout the body helps the therapist localize pathological problems (Upledger and Vrodevoogd, 1983).

Valuable information is thus gained through the evaluation of the craniosacral motion by evaluating its rate, amplitude, symmetry, and quality (flexion/extension) (Burget, 2002). In the optimal healthy individual, these qualities are regular and rhythmic and can be felt by the therapist to be occurring six to twelve times per minute. With good palpatory skills, these rhythms can be felt easily through the head and sacrum as well as throughout the entire body (Smoley, 1991).

It is imperative to understand that pressure and/or tension can be transmitted throughout the skull and brain from restrictions in the spine, extremities, or anywhere within the peripheral tissues because the connective tissue is continuous. Thus, a restriction anywhere in the body can create tensile forces that contract and compress the brain and spinal cord due to pressures applied within the dural tube.

THE PHILOSOPHY BEHIND
CRANIOSACRAL THERAPY

Generally speaking, people want good health and abundant energy to be able to start and complete those tasks that are meaningful to them. They yearn to be competent, creative, and compassionate, and to be able to both give and receive the respect they deserve. People wish for personal freedom, to choose for themselves what is most important to them, the direction they will take in life, and with which friends and lovers they will share their lives. Simply by being human, one craves to bring about healthy change in his or her life and to work through areas that are not working out so well. People desire to learn to be more fully human and alive in working through their experiences while becoming more fully aware of their relationships, their world, and themselves (Nolen-Hoeksema and Davis, 2002). They aspire to deepen their understanding of themselves and to develop and define more precisely the expression of their own lives in order to fully realize their humanity and accept both its beauty and its pain.

It is often physical pain that causes a person to become involved in craniosacral therapy. This therapeutic modality can be an excellent treatment to move one through and beyond bodily pain and restore physiological function. Pain is usually a very good motivator for people to start searching for a better way of existing (Nolen-Hoeksema and Davis, 2002). Why else would one even want to change? Craniosacral therapy, thus, can bring about a renaissance of change in every aspect of a person's being. It can work through one's physical pain and dysfunctions and bring about unimaginable opportunities for realization of mind/body health and a long overdue upliftment of the battered human spirit (Hutch, 2000; Wethington, 2003).

One reason that craniosacral treatment can be effective is that the combination of techniques can enervate enough change, movement, and energy to break through a captive's physical barriers and psychological entropy. It can change the status quo enough to move them on to a new plane of awareness in which they can become self-empowered and have choice (Persaud, 2002). Any change in the physiological state is accompanied by a corresponding change in the cognitive-emotional state, whether it is conscious or unconscious; and inversely, every change in the cognitive-emotional state, conscious or unconscious, is accompanied by a corresponding change in the physiological state (Heinrich, 1991a). Many ways, places, and therapies are available to turn to when individuals cannot find their way anymore. Many gifted therapists, body workers, psychologists, ministers, and doctors are available to help patients get back on their path of healing and wholeness. Just as many spokes support and strengthen a wheel, each reaching for the internal center or core, many ways and modalities exist for the patient to turn to for help. Many processes for healing the body and mind can come through modalities and therapies from the traditional allopathic medical model. Craniosacral therapy is just one of such modalities.

The craniosacral therapy practitioner essentially helps the body release restrictions that a person has been unable to overcome on their own. This approach is not only gentle but the method is extremely safe and effective, allowing the body's normal, self-correcting tendencies to heal the real problems (Smoley, 1991; Upledger and Vredevoogd, 1983). Craniosacral therapy can help heal the body, mind, and spirit. It is truly a powerful way to work through transformation. It helps the body, mind, and soul of a person to find its way back from wherever it has been lost or discarded—to find its way back home to a life that is more meaningful, integrated, and unrestricted (Heinrich, 1989).

Craniosacral therapy, thus, can help individuals unravel their lives by moving them through their barriers and pains and bringing them back into their wholeness. It is a potent tool that can assist those who are broken and very injured (Nolen-Hoeksema and Davis, 2002). In addition, it can be a tool for those who are quite far along on the path of self-actualization to fine-tune and move even further into transformation. As one heals he or she is led to increased awareness and a quieter mind. Healing enhances one's natural tendency to seek out order in all areas of life, moving from chaos and drama to a life of meaning and purpose (Nolen-Hoeksema and Davis, 2002; Hutch, 2000). One can find simplicity and peace in what used to be utterly baffling. Anger and resentments, although justified, can melt into forgiveness and ultimate acceptance of the past (West, 2001). One can find answers and acceptance where only contempt and conflict had been. Thus, through such therapies, individuals will find more order and balance in their internal lives, which will bring order and transformation into their external life. In order to grow/transform, one has to let go of fears, walls, and failings. He or she must change. Craniosacral therapy, through a caring and competent therapist, can help a person do exactly that (Bodeau, 2002).

THE CRANIOSACRAL THERAPEUTIC PROCESS

Craniosacral therapy helps bridge the gap between body workers and mind workers. Craniosacral therapy is based on the principle that the body really does know exactly how to heal itself. When a person receives craniosacral therapy, he or she is basically using a facilitator to encourage the body to let go of that which is no longer necessary (Gerome, 1997; Smoley, 1991).

Craniosacral therapy is a very gentle manual therapeutic technique. In fact, at times the person being treated may not even feel what is happening except at a subconscious level. It is a gentle, hands-on therapy that requires compassionate and understanding therapists who are able to create a relationship of trust and cooperation between themselves and their patients (Upledger and Vredevoogd, 1983). It is a treatment modality that is best used by properly trained therapists to examine and treat or release restrictions anywhere within the body (Glaser, 2002). A restriction can be an adhesion/scarring or an energy block anywhere within the body. In therapy, both the therapist and the patient are working together toward the goal of release and freedom from pain for the patient. Release relies largely on the patient's own process to remove obstacles. People cannot be forced to move beyond their own ability to let go. Free will and personal control is the bottom line. The therapist only facilitates the process with encouragement and support (Smoley, 1991).

Unlike other forms of allopathic medicine, the therapist does not dictate how the correction should be made (Upledger and Vredevoogd, 1983). There is no cookbook or set process for treatments. Both the therapist and the patient are there to discover together how the correction can best be made. Therapists must follow where the patient's body brings them. The release will come only in its own way. The patient's body knows how to move through its barriers toward self-correction. With the therapist's help, the patient's body will find its own resolve to the internal problems and imbalance. Both the therapist and patient must wait, respect, follow, encourage, and support the process and each other. It is sometimes very difficult to accept this process. The therapist may literally sit on one of the patient's restrictions through several treatments before the patient is ready to let it go and move forward (Burget, 2002). It is within the patient's domain and not the therapist's when progress is made (Hutch, 2000). Sometimes visual imagery can be a beneficial tool to help patients become more aware of their barriers and to help them work through the process (Gerome, 1997). Color imagery is especially helpful for patients to visualize and release within the therapy session.

To help a person understand how craniosacral therapy works, it is important to understand the connective tissue and fascia of the body. The fascia is a tough connective tissue that literally holds one's body together. It runs similar to a mesh or sheath that surrounds and divides every structure within the body. The tiniest nerve has its own connective tissue sheath or envelope, as does the largest of the organs and bones. In fact, about half of the muscular attachments of the body are to fascia. The fascia is a continuous "body stocking" lying under the skin (Reuben, 1987). It can be described as tubes within tubes. It is there to separate and support every structure in one's body. Connective tissue is made up of very small collagen fibers, which form the mesh. The majority of these fibers run longitudinally through the body. Transverse facial plains run across our bodies horizontally that act architecturally similar to floors in a building, separating organ systems and offering additional support for the body (so that it can be held vertically in space against the forces of gravity). These floors are the diaphragms of the body, such as the pelvic floor, the respiratory diaphragm, the thoracic outlet, the occipital cranial base, and the tentorium cerebelli. The fascial system is a complete and single system, reaching from the uppermost region of the internal cranium to the base of the feet, creating a three-dimensional web. This is important to know to fully understand craniosacral therapy (Barnes, 1990).

Think for a moment about the way the body heals following a trauma, whether it is physical or psychological. As the body tries to recover from insult, injury, or unabated stress, the body will lay down thousands of collagen fibers where it is injured or inflamed. A swelling process in our bodies always brings in these fibers. The body initially tries to heal itself in this way. The body in its natural healing mode will lay down these fibers or connective tissue to ultimately form adhesions. As a protective mechanism, the body will do this in areas of stress or trauma to enhance structure, reduce bleeding, or wall off areas of infection or swelling. This new collagen formation laid down after trauma will then begin to distort the inherent collagen web that surrounds every structure within the body.

Unfortunately, collagen has an inherent quality of shrinking over time. This occurs externally in persons who may have suffered severe burns. For example, the distortions and disfigurement that can be produced from this shrinking of the connective tissue can be seen in the physical distortions of a face and its features that have been badly burned. This shrinking, which naturally occurs within the collagen web, will ultimately lead to a reduction in tissue mobility, fluid exchange, and health because it causes compression and tension on and through life-giving structures and organs. Where connective tissue has become denser or is compressing organs in the body, dysfunction will follow. Those denser tissues are then not able to function properly, leading to devastating physical compromise and loss of health. Where this internal connective tissue web has been affected or bound, organs and structures can become diseased or compromised through the loss of efficient circulation. Such density or restriction does not allow these bound or compressed tissues optimal oxygenation nor removal of metabolic wastes and toxins. The density compromises the function of one's cells and, ultimately, one's health. The restricted tissues will not allow the fluids of the body to move to their optimum efficiency, not only affecting the amount of oxygen brought to the tissues but the exchange of hormones, enzymes, neurotransmitters, neuromodulators, and neuropeptides (including but not limited to endorphins, serotonin, dynorphins, enkephalins, acetylcholine, and dopamine).

Craniosacral therapy can be used to treat problems of pain and dysfunction throughout the entire body where patients may have sustained injury through emotional or physical trauma, vascular bleeds, surgery, infection, or swelling. These are all areas where connective tissue has been laid down in excess and where the beautiful collagen web has become distorted (Upledger and Vredevoogd, 1983).

Chronic overarousal, emotional distress, depression, and anxiety can lead to organic damage through inflammation and fibrosis in many areas of our bodies. For example, we are all aware of how stress can lead to heart disease, colitis, and ulcers. Events such as abuse, neglect, insult, and injury can become frozen in our bodies. This is called tissue memory. The patient, thus, needs to look at himself or herself as a total integration among spirit, mind, and body (Cox, 2002). Craniosacral therapy is one means in which to accomplish this.

Outwardly, the treatment can seem very passive and uneventful. It may look as if the therapist is not doing anything other than resting his or her hands on the patient. The patient (in his or her internal environment) may or may not be aware of large or subtle shifts and changes occurring within his or her body.

Craniosacral therapy is an effective evaluation tool and treatment modality. Skilled therapists can monitor the craniosacral rhythm readily and easily pinpoint the source of an obstruction or restriction. Once the source of restriction has been determined, therapists can assist with the natural movement of fluid and related soft tissue to help their patients' bodies self-correct. Therapists usually do not apply any more than five grams of pressure to the system, making craniosacral therapy a very subtle but effective noninvasive tool to help those who have suffered insults to their body (Upledger and Vredevoogd, 1983). Therapists will most often use very passive palpation and utilize only very light pressure, as if their hand was a leaf floating on the water. If the therapist applies excessive pressure, neuromuscular defenses in the patient may be activated, and the intended results may not occur. The body has a wide spectrum of different tissue densities containing hard tissues such as bone and soft tissues such as muscles and organs. The therapist must develop excellent palpatory skills that will inform him or her when the treatments are effective with an osseous or a membranous restriction and how a release feels. To become an effective therapist, one must be able to feel membrane tension patterns, fluid wave patterns, and subtle energy (Cohen, 1989a).

The craniosacral rhythm is a unifying wave pattern utilizing the entire spectrum of densities. Therapists must learn to trust themselves and to feel these very subtle differences. Therapists listen to the body through palpations or kinesthetic skills, and then allow or introduce gentle traction compression or lifting (Cohen, 1989b,c). If a therapist encounters resistance, it may indicate an underlying restriction. Continuous light traction will usually release these restrictions. Deep breathing by the patient can also assist in the release of resistant restrictions. As the restriction releases, the therapist will feel a change and will feel the elastic recoil of the tissue dissipate. This signifies that the release is complete. *Release* is the term applied to the sense of softening and relaxation that is perceptible when the technique has come to a successful completion (Upledger and Vredevoogd, 1983). The therapist cannot dictate how the correction is to be made but only assists the patient's body with its own natural, self-corrective activities. This gentle, noninvasive approach ensures that no serious errors or side effects will occur, because the patient's craniosacral system itself decides how the correction will be accomplished. The therapist simply helps remove the obstacles and activate/empower the patient for change.

Therapists must "blend" with their patients and be extremely reverent in their touch, utilizing kinesthetic or proproceptive senses of their own body to guide them through their patients' body. Therapists use their hand on the surface to feel for fluid waveforms, pressure, and membrane tension (Cohen, 1989a). The blended hand is fluid in character and becomes fully sensory; it only needs to ride with the wave pattern of the patient. Passive palpation is required so that the movement can be felt and evaluated throughout the patient's entire body (since the body is an enclosed fibromembranous sack from the top of the head to the distal toes) (Cohen, 1989b). Once a source of restriction has been determined, a therapist can assist the natural movement of the fluid and related soft tissue to help the body self-correct (Smoley, 1991).

Asymmetry with the rhythm will show the therapist where the problems are located (Reuben, 1987). In most cases, restoration of the symmetry in the area of restriction will bring about release and healing. The examiner is limited only by his or her palpatory skills and knowledge of anatomy. It is this knowledge that will help the therapist locate the problems. It is important for the therapist to be in tune with the patient and to be completely nonthreatening. The patient will be better able to relax and more open to release. Release is always a positive event in the restoration of physical, emotional, behavioral, and cognitive function.

Dysfunctions or pathology can be felt and removed anywhere within the body by holding the craniosacral movement against the hydraulic pressure created by the ventricles. The therapist merely gently holds the body from this inherent movement for several phases of the craniosacral rhythm, and the restrictions release and resolve themselves, clearing the body from these anchoring forces. The therapist and sometimes the patient will feel a pulsing or wobbling sensation just preceding a major release or shift (Upledger and Vredevoogd, 1983). The patient will often feel a softening, warming, or lengthening of tissues that previously felt dense, tight, and possibly painful. Remember, the body is always trying to find its own homeostasis and, with craniosacral treatment, one is utilizing the patient's natural self-corrective physiological activities. The therapist's light touch will assist the hydraulic forces inherent in the body to improve its own natural internal environment. Self-corrections are the key to lasting changes in the body, just as self-knowledge brings about freedom, choice, and life enhancement (Nolen-Hoeksema and Davis, 2002). Release is the culmination of relaxation of the nervous reflexes that may have been causing increased tone in the body. In addition, a lengthening of the restricted tissues back to their original dimensions can occur.

Tissue trauma memory is also extremely important in this therapeutic process. Many times patients will discuss their trauma in great detail—where they were, who was with them, how old they were at the time of the insult, the color of the room they were in, smells involved, etc.—all that was present at the time of their injuries. The deeper patients are able to go into the therapeutic process, the more they are able to get into these memories. Such a process seems to enable patients to both remember and relive (to some extent) the traumatic, anxiety-provoking event while ultimately bringing about healing (Gerome, 1997).

As outlined in Exhibit 9.1, craniosacral therapy can be appropriate and beneficial for many medical conditions. Only a few situations exist in which craniosacral therapy would be contraindicated. Contraindications include conditions in which a variation and/or slight increase in intracranial pressure could cause instability, such as an acute aneurysm, a recent intracranial hemorrhage or cerebrovascular accident, or if a patient has a preexisting severe bleeding disorder that could result in hemorrhage. Craniosacral therapy should never be used during acute stages of stroke or head injury (Burget, 2002).

**EXHIBIT 9.1. Indications for the use
of craniosacral therapy.**

Traumatic brain injury
Central nervous system disorders
Migraine headaches
Chronic neck and back pain
Emotional difficulties
Motor-coordination impairments
Stress- and tension-related disorders
Temporomandibular joint dysfunctions
Orthopedic problems
Chronic fatigue
Scoliosis
Neurovascular disorders
Immune disorders
Infantile disorders
Colic
Post-traumatic stress disorder
Autism
Postsurgical dysfunctions
Learning disabilities
Fibromyalgia and other connective-tissue disorders

GOALS AND USE OF CRANIOSACRAL THERAPY
WITH BRAIN-INJURED PATIENTS

The following is a list of therapeutic goals of craniosacral therapy with brain-injured clients:

1. To relieve pressure, compression, and torque from shrinking adhesions that resulted from their injuries affecting the brain and other vital organs and tissues
2. To enhance the exchange of body fluids such as blood, lymph, cerebrospinal fluid, hormones, and neurotransmitters to enhance general health
3. To assist the body in carrying away old metabolites, toxins, and pathogens that may be hampering good health
4. To improve behavioral control and reduce aggressiveness, agitation, and anger
5. To enhance motivation and spontaneity and reduce depression
6. To enhance functional and optimal movement patterns
7. To enhance cognitive function and academic achievement
8. To enhance the restoration of good physical alignment, posture, comfort, and function
9. To relieve chronic pain issues from which TBI (traumatic brain injury) survivors commonly suffer
10. To reduce the frequency of seizures
11. To enhance optimal sleep hygiene by helping TBI survivors sleep more soundly
12. To help TBI survivors find emotional and physical comfort within themselves
13. To enhance interpersonal relationships
14. To enhance parasympathetic tone by assisting TBI survivors in relaxation
15. To produce an overall quieting of the nervous system
16. To reduce post-traumatic stress disorder symptoms such as anxiety, nervousness, apprehension, social withdrawal, phobic reactions, muscle tension, irritability, startle reactions, impaired concentration, and repetitive nightmares
17. To minimize reliance on medications whenever possible to reduce the potential of drug interactions and side effects

Craniosacral therapy is a very effective method of releasing the remains of old traumas (from any source) and restoring healthy functioning throughout the body (Upledger and Vredevoogd, 1983). Following a brain injury, some of the brain cells will die and other cells will be affected from the scarring. Brain injury survivors often are not able to function at their full potential until the scarring is released. The object of craniosacral therapy in such cases is to bring back the cells/tissues that have been compromised but are still alive to their optimum ability to function. Craniosacral therapy (anywhere in the body) can enhance the internal environment that surrounds the brain and spinal cord. When something goes awry within one's body, the brain and spinal cord often suffer due to abnormal stresses such as torque, compression, loss of full oxygenation, loss of full toxin or metabolic waste removal, and general loss of full metabolic and immunological fluid exchange. An injury or imbalance within the craniosacral system or anywhere within the body can adversely affect the nervous system via scarring and by reducing its proper function. Such traumas can cause sensory, motor, cognitive, behavioral, and neurological disabilities.

Since the brain and the spinal cord are the core of one's physical being, the role of the craniosacral system in the development and performance of the brain and spinal cord is a vital one. An imbalance or dysfunction in the craniosacral system could lead to only a slight impairment in one's neurological function or could cause profound sensory, motor, and neurological disabilities. If the brain and spinal cord are not able to function optimally, one's senses, emotions, behaviors, and motor functions will not work optimally. Craniosacral therapy, thus, can be a very effective method of both examination and treatment devised to correct problems throughout the entire body that have resulted from the brain injury.

Craniosacral treatments facilitate better tissue mobility throughout the body (including the brain) which can lead to enhanced blood circulation and fluid exchange throughout all of the tissues released. Body fluids such as blood, cerebrospinal fluid, and lymph are able to enhance oxygenation and removal of metabolic wastes, pathogens, and toxins as well as enhancing hormone and neurotransmitter exchange throughout the body. Proper treatment enhances sensory, motor, behavioral, and intellectual functions (Upledger, 1978; Reuben, 1987).

If any procedure or accident "jams" the cranial sutures, a person can lose the normal blood flow in the cranium, affecting the brain. This could result from a forceps delivery for a newborn, a car accident causing a brain injury, a fall on the tailbone or sacrum, a sports injury, or even a misfortunate dental procedure (Reuben, 1987). This jamming of the cranial bones can create pain and malfunctions in many different bodily systems. One result of such trauma is irritation of the brain, which can lead to many problems for the injured person (including hyperkinetic behaviors) (Reuben, 1987). When a trained therapist alleviates the pressure from the jammed cranial bones of a brain-injured patient through craniosacral treatment, the hyperkinesias can sometimes disappear within two to three minutes (Reuben, 1987). However, not all hyperkinetic behaviors come from problems within the craniosacral system but may be a result of food allergies, chemical intolerances, or emotional/psychological problems (Reuben, 1987).

Persons suffering from traumatic brain injury often suffer from anxiety and disappointment in many areas of their life. Self-esteem, cognitive performance, home life, and relationships with friends and family often suffer. In general, their daily experiences can be littered with tension, loneliness, and failure (Linley and Joseph, 2003). It only makes sense that as brain function is improved, cognitive function would also improve. Through therapy, patients begin the process of healing, and are able to think more clearly, stay more focused, and make better choices. As the body and mind are influenced positively through the release of restrictions, the patient will find that interpersonal relationships improve and that cognitive, behavioral, and emotional functioning also improve (Upledger, 1978, 1983).

Chronic Pain

Many of the TBI patients seen for treatment suffer from chronic pain issues related to their accidents and trauma. Many have suffered from severe orthopedic as well as neurological injuries throughout their bodies. It is common for these patients to complain of such symptoms as reoccurring severe headaches or back problems (Sims, 1989; Upledger and Vredevoogd, 1983; Danese, 1989). Many TBI patients suffer from restrictions in their movement and structural alignment problems. Craniosacral therapy has been a wonderful modality for helping with these issues. Therapy assists patients in revitalizing the central nervous system as well as releasing restrictions throughout the body that have contributed to many kinds of physical dysfunctions and pain. Positive structural-alignment changes result in profound significant improvements in pain control or reduction.

Trauma-Induced Seizure Disorders

Some craniosacral therapists have been reluctant to work with people who suffer from seizure disorders. However, craniosacral therapy is gentle and noninvasive and uses only the patient's body's wisdom to find balance, thus therapists can be assured that such treatments will not cause harm. Craniosacral therapy has been known to completely relieve seizures in some cases, or at worst have a neutral effect on the incidence of seizures in such patients (Upledger, 1996).

Trauma-Induced Sleep Disorders

According to sleep researchers, the average adult needs between eight to nine hours of sleep per night to function optimally. It has been found that most people get only seven hours of sleep per night on average. Sleep problems are quite prevalent in people who have suffered brain injury, resulting in the patient feeling tired even after ten hours of sleep. It is not uncommon for them to feel tired throughout the day, especially during the post-TBI recovery period. These patients find it difficult to fall asleep, and they may wake several times each night, which further hampers the desired restorative effects of sleep. Sleep problems can often be a "weak link" in optimal functioning. Sleep problems not only affect mood, cognition, and general performance, but also affect the metabolic, cardiovascular, and immune functions. The circadian rhythms of sleep are essential for maintaining optimal health. These rhythms control the timing of variations in body temperature, cardiovascular rates, secretion of melatonin in the pineal gland, and levels of prolactin and growth hormone in the pituitary and cortisol in the adrenal gland. Craniosacral therapy can help a person to restore his or her own optimal circadian rhythms.

Such therapies can enhance the parasympathetic nervous system, which can affect sleep function.

Self-Depression and Negative Self-Concept

As previously discussed in this chapter, times occur when a person needs help in realizing balance and freedom. It is important for a person to accept the darker sides of himself or herself (West, 2001). This process is even more difficult for people who have suffered a brain injury, since they may feel as if they have lost everything and may never be able to "fit in" again (Linley and Joseph, 2003; Wethington, 2003). However, the more one is able to practice self-love and forgiveness the more he or she is able to love and forgive others. This will always bring more balance and improved relationships into one's life and restore one's sense of belonging (West, 2001). Loneliness seems to be one of the most painful experiences for persons who have suffered brain injury. Via craniosacral therapy, therapists are often able to help their brain-injured patients let go and find peace within themselves and in the world around them. Therapy helps the autonomic nervous system balance the parasympathetic nervous system and the now hyperactive sympathetic nervous system. Therapists often observe their patients taking in a deep breath or sigh as they progress in treatment. Negative patterns that are held and that often keep the body in poor alignment often melt away. As therapy progresses, patients will find more comfort and will feel as if they are able to breathe deeper with greater ease.

Other Medical/Physical Conditions

Craniosacral therapy can also be extremely effective in assisting patients to better manage stress-related disorders. Symptoms such as fatigue, headaches, poor digestion, anxiety, and temporomandibular joint dysfunctions are just a few areas that respond favorably to treatment (Sims, 1989; Heinrich, 1991a,b). Craniosacral therapy works to reverse the debilitating effects of stress by providing the conditions in which the nervous system can rest and rejuvenate. Other conditions for which craniosacral therapy has proven effective are various sensory disorders, such as eye–motor coordination problems, dyslexia, loss of taste or smell, tinnitus, vertigo, and neuralgias such as sciatica.

PTSD

Post-traumatic stress disorder (PTSD) has traditionally been difficult to treat, and many people with brain injury suffer from this disorder. It is recognized as a condition that can result from any traumatic
experience—not just those occurring on the battlefield (Modlin,
1986). Craniosacral therapy has been found to be an excellent tool to
help release traumatic memories and relieve the tension and pain associated with the traumas (Gerome, 1997). Anxiety, irritability, startle reactions, impaired concentration, and repetitive nightmares are
often reduced in frequency and intensity via treatment. Sometimes
these symptoms are totally eliminated.

Often when a TBI survivor's life is falling apart, it is difficult for
them to put what is happening into perspective (Workman, 2002). In
addition to their cognitive impairments, which interfere with their
ability to understand what is happening to them, patients often suffer
from agnosia due to the injuries. As discussed elsewhere in this text,
agnosia is a condition brought on by the brain injury itself that may
make it impossible for the patient to understand his or her deficits.
Such patients believe that they are functioning as they have always
functioned even though it is evident to their families, friends, and
peers that they are not. Agnosia is a severe condition that limits the
patient's insight into what is happening and interferes with internal
motivation to change in ways that would be of benefit. Agnosia can at
times lead the patient into having little to no desire to change nor any
sense of a need to change. Agnosia is often one of the biggest challenges for a TBI survivor to overcome.

The therapist can use craniosacral treatment to reduce or resolve
physical pain and assist the TBI survivor in releasing the negative patterns that affect all areas of their lives. Most often, syndromes that
have both psychological and physical components respond best to
self-awareness and responsibility by the patients, but such awareness
may not be possible after brain injury. However, even in patients with
such an agnosia, physical pain can be used as a motivator for them to
participate in and progress via therapy. The great benefit of craniosacral therapy in such cases is that treatments can help patients
improve all aspects of their life. As their physical pain decreases, a
corresponding improvement in behaviors and enhanced cognitive
functioning often occurs. However, therapists can only kindly and

gently guide their patients to examine any problematic emotions such as anger, resentment, or stress. The patients that are able to receive the most benefit from their treatments are those that are able to work well with their therapist. Thus, the therapist needs to continually enhance cooperation in and understanding of the therapeutic process (Upledger, 1983). This often occurs over time as the therapist builds rapport and helps their patient move through the physical pain.

STRUCTURE AND USE OF CRANIOSACRAL THERAPY IN A HOSPITAL-BASED TBI REHABILITATION PROGRAM

Although craniosacral therapy is often provided in outpatient clinics and private practices, it can be quite beneficial for patients with traumatic brain injury who have associated neurobehavioral dysfunctions (Upledger and Karni, 1979b; Upledger, 1980). In such cases, an application of craniosacral therapy within a multidisciplinary or interdisciplinary treatment will be the most effective. In such cases and settings, primary issues typically to be addressed with craniosacral therapy can include physical, emotional/psychological, cognitive, and behavioral dysfunction (Upledger, 1980). Thus, many issues may surface in one or more of these areas, requiring involvement by other team members in such professions as neurology/physiatry, psychiatry/psychology, speech therapy, occupational therapy, rehabilitation nursing, and behavioral psychology. Ideally, a craniosacral therapist will meet with the treatment team at least weekly (if not more) and/or meet with professionals on an individual basis as needed as discipline-specific issues arise. Goals, barriers, or problems and progress should be ultimately discussed among the team members and addressed from a holistic perspective. The ideal situation in such a program is to have all team members (which includes the patient and family members) accept and collectively work on treatment goals that are appropriate to the individual patient.

The therapist will find it best to begin the craniosacral evaluation with a comprehensive physical therapy assessment. This evaluation process includes the following three steps:

1. Examine the whole body, evaluating the patient's posture and assessing for even small deviations.
2. Assess the patient's biomechanics and functional movement (such as how the patient walks and generally how he or she moves).
3. Evaluate the patient's muscle tone, range of motion, balance, joint mobility, strength, pain level and locations, and sleep patterns.

Some specific assessment methods include the following:

• Watch how patients get on the treatment table and how their bodies position themselves while relaxing.
• Look for areas where patients are unable to relax and even how they are breathing. Factors such as weakness, tightness, or restriction of motion are noted for later consideration in the treatment plan.
• Test the dural tube to rule out restrictions in the craniosacral complex that may be causing pain or are transferring tension or pressure from other sources.
• Observe closely the way patients move, the way they stand, how they function, and where their pain patterns are.
• Have patients rate their pain using the pain scale of 0 to 10. Break down each complaint area and ask how it feels when it is at its best, how it feels normally, and how much pain they have when it is at its worst.

When reviewing sleep patterns, determine when the patient encounters sleep difficulties during the night; for example, is it when trying to fall asleep or is it a problem of waking throughout the night? Is the patient lying awake for hours? How does he or she feel after a night's sleep? Does the patient wake refreshed, or feel as if he or she has worked all night long?

A comprehensive evaluation of the patient's posture can provide the therapist with critical information regarding where the restrictions exist within the body. Continuous reevaluation should occur as treatment progresses since restrictions will change over time and will continue to reveal where to work next.

Craniosacral treatment is best done in a quiet, safe room in which the patient is to lie down and completely relax (Breggin, 2002). The therapist will typically have the patient lie supine while on the treatment table, with the therapist sitting on a moveable chair at the head of the table. A soft pillow is placed under the patient's cervical spine to enhance the best cervical alignment and relaxation possible. In addition, pillows are placed under the knees to take pressure off of the low back. This is extremely important, specifically for patients who suffer from back problems.

The more comfortable the brain-injured patient is during treatment, the more he or she will be able to release restriction and heal. During the session it will be necessary for the therapist to move to various areas around the table such as beside the torso, arms, legs, or feet. The therapist will often cradle the patient's arm or leg at times so that the extremity can literally float without the pull of gravity. The therapist will need to sustain a posture for the patient until he or she is able to release the barrier. Soft background music is often used to enhance the patient's ability to relax. As discussed in detail in Chapter 4, music will sometimes help the patient to better tune into the internal landscape. Music also helps center energy and awareness inward. The therapist should always encourage relaxation, comfort, respect, and trust to enhance the patients' ability to reach the point at which they are able to let go (Breggin, 2002).

The patient is able to stay fully clothed during treatment, which is another advantage of craniosacral therapy, especially for the brain-injured patient (Upledger, 1997). This is especially helpful if the patient has sexual-abuse issues or is self-conscious about his or her physical appearance. It is crucial that the patient be kept warm during treatment to decrease physical stress and enhance release. The added insulation from a blanket seems to help those patients who may have suffered from physical or sexual abuse in their lives to be able to relax and release more easily.

TBI patients typically enjoy craniosacral treatment and find it very relaxing. It is usually a positive experience for them and they will often request this treatment when they see the therapist. It may be the first time in their lives since the injury that they have experienced touch that wasn't threatening or painful, and this can enhance their self-acceptance and self-love while reducing maladaptive behaviors

(Breggin, 2002). Periodically, a therapist will come upon a patient who finds it hard to be touched or to even lie still on a treatment table. In such cases, the therapist can first provide treatments for very short intervals. Soon the patient will be wanting to lie on the table for however long it takes to complete a treatment. Just as each TBI patient is unique, each patient will experience craniosacral sessions differently. The immediate results will be diverse. One patient may be very relaxed and fall asleep during the treatment and may even want to sleep for hours after a session (Upledger, 1996). Others may experience an increase in energy. Pain may also increase for short periods during the treatment and the patient may need to be encouraged to endure until the pain improves. Reduction in pain can be immediate, or it may improve gradually over time. As mentioned before, some patients will remember forgotten incidents while being treated or even following treatment (Gerome, 1997). Memories can surface in dreams or images. The therapist and other professionals, such as rehabilitation psychologists, can assist the patient during this process.

The quality of consciousness or the enhancement of awareness for the patient is usually proportional to the amount of repressed fearful material that is brought up from the unconscious. These unconscious memories will often come to the surface to be confronted and resolved with the therapist and other treatment team members. Through this therapeutic process, the patient will finally be able to put these traumas into perspective, to find understanding, and to work toward forgiveness where it is needed to help restore his or her life (West, 2001).

Much effort with the TBI patient may be put forth before a flash of insight is brought about. The therapist may have to work with the patient on the same restriction for a long period of time or over many treatments (Burget, 2002). The patient may just not be ready to face the change. Following a treatment, the patient may feel very physically drained and tired, or may experience increased energy and stamina. Reduction of pain and an increase in function may come about immediately or it may come gradually over several treatments and days. It may also take time to reorganize the body following some large releases. At times the patient will feel achy following treatment, and old pains may be brought to the surface. This is called a healing crisis. In such cases, therapists may need to reassure their patients about the pains that may come up so that they do not become overly concerned or frightened.

The number of treatments needed will vary widely for the TBI patient depending on the condition of the patient being treated. It can range from just one treatment to several treatments a week for many weeks or months. A treatment will usually last about forty-five minutes to an hour and sometimes even longer. Some treatments may need to be shortened for patients who are just beginning treatment. However, as treatment progresses, patients' comfort levels will increase as will their ability to endure longer sessions. It takes time to resolve areas that have been compromised for a long time.

Because craniosacral therapy helps the body resume its natural healing processes, it is common for improvements to continue even weeks after a session. Some patients may need time for reorganization as the body adapts to the releases from previously held patterns. They may need reassurance that this is normal. The therapist should reassure patients that even though what they may be experiencing is painful or doesn't feel good, it is actually a positive sign that their bodies are releasing old toxins, tissue memory, and old patterns, and that they are finding a new way to move (Linley and Joseph, 2003).

CASE EXAMPLE

Tom B. was a twenty-four-year-old male who suffered a traumatic brain injury when he was eighteen years old. He was a senior in high school at the time of his injury. He was involved in a motor vehicle accident while with his then girlfriend. Since the injury Tom had been suffering from severe behavioral difficulties, such as physical aggression, self-injurious behaviors, sexually inappropriate behaviors, and property destruction. He was finding it very difficult to accept what had happened to him and just wanted to be the way he was before his accident. He also suffered from severe physical disabilities. He had left hemiparesis and suffered from ataxia on the left side of his body. His left leg was internally rotated and flexed, and he would limp and drag his left leg while walking. He held his left arm in a tightly flexed spastic pattern against his chest. He was not able to use this arm functionally at all. He was frustrated by his physical disabilities and was depressed and anxious.

He didn't know how to handle his anger or frustration, which often manifested as aggression toward himself or others (or by "trashing" his room and the unit). He also suffered from severe headaches that occurred at least once a week. Because of his anger and aggression he found it difficult to maintain relationships with his family and old friends. His ties with his loved ones were severed or greatly impaired. He was lonely and frustrated. He had difficulty relating to his peers and would use physically threatening gestures to get them to do what he wanted. He was verbally aggressive and sexually inappropriate with the staff. He had difficulty falling asleep and would wake three to four times each night.

Working with Tom was intense. He received physical therapy two to three times per week and received craniosacral therapy for about nine months. He had a comprehensive holistic program, utilizing all of the services the rehabilitation facility offered. The neurologist worked with Tom through all of his pharmacological needs. The behavior analysts created a positive behavioral modification program that was successful for him.

Tom progressed slowly but surely, and he found many benefits through his holistic treatment. He became more calm and self-accepting. He was able to think before acting and his life started coming back into his control. He was no longer aggressive with his peers or the staff who worked with him. He was no longer sexually inappropriate. When he left the rehabilitation center, he no longer suffered from ataxia on the left side of his body and he was able to use his left arm functionally. The arm was no longer pulled up into the spastic pattern but was comfortably positioned at his side. He could use it as he willed. He walked almost normally, having only a very slight limp. The internal rotation, flexion pattern that he held in his left lower extremity was completely resolved. He no longer suffered from headaches and was able to sleep throughout the night. His anxiety and depression lessened. His relationship with his family was also starting to improve. He was getting along better with his peers and his angry outbursts with aggression against others were totally eliminated. He learned how to manage his anger in more appropriate ways, and he no longer injured himself or "trashed" the unit when he became frustrated. It took some time, but Tom was a great success story. His life and self-esteem were restored, he was able to come to terms with what had happened to him, and he found much more peace and contentment in his life.

APPENDIX:
TRAINING AND EDUCATIONAL RESOURCES

Professional Training, Certification, and Organizations for Craniosacral Therapy

To become a competent craniosacral therapist, one needs to realize that it is impossible to fully understand craniosacral work from reading and studying books or even from attending all of the recommended workshops.

Multiple techniques must be learned, and many subtle skills and kinesthetic perceptions must be mastered. Craniosacral therapy is not only a science but an art form. It is truly a healing modality. Craniosacral therapists are first trained, licensed health care practitioners. Competence in craniosacral therapy requires years of practice, unending compassion, trust, and humility. It often takes years of experience in working with patients to gain a level of competency in craniosacral technique.

What is anatomically, physiologically, and scientifically known or experienced must become integrated as the therapist arrives at the point at which the distinction between facts and skills is dissolved. Therapists use their intellect but ultimately must learn to trust their hands and perceptions. They must believe the information that is received during the treatment process. It is at this point that craniosacral therapy becomes not only a science but also an art form. With this approach to treatment the therapist is able to learn a significant amount about the patient. The therapist has to have a pure intention of being of assistance to the patient to heal (Upledger, 1996).

Therapists are trained to detect tiny variations in movement as well as to perform techniques that will free up the flow of bodily fluids. The work requires great sensitivity and respect for the body's inherent wisdom. Although certain conditions or diseases create similar patterns, each person is unique in how his or her body needs to be treated. This will be revealed as one works with many patients.

Several qualities are necessary to become competent in craniosacral therapy. These qualities include excellent listening skills and the ability to blend with the patient and the process. Therapists need to be aware of their own issues and not let them become confused with their patients' (Breggin, 2002). Patients will consciously or unconsciously try to move the therapist away from their own issues that they are afraid to confront/address. Competent therapists are able to identify their patients' defenses and resistance maneuvers. Therapists must learn to extract and understand the purposes of defenses and work with them and not against them. The therapist will also need to identify with and encourage the parts of the patient that truly desire resolution and wholeness. The therapist must develop an ability to help discharge negative emotions and energies to help the patient convert these to something more positive (Rizzuto, 2003; Hutch, 2000).

A primary training site for craniosacral therapy is the Upledger Institute in Palm Beach Gardens, Florida. Acceptance for attendance at Upledger Institute workshops is based on the applicant's background, training, and interests. The Upledger Institute encourages licensed health care practitioners that wish to participate in education to view craniosacral therapy as an adjunctive modality to be integrated into an existing discipline, such as physical therapy. The Institute may make exceptions to this policy as appropriate.

They may waive the requirement of being a health care professional for family members or caregivers who they feel could help a child, parent, or relative via the use of craniosacral therapy. Other special cases may involve potential referral persons such as schoolteachers, administrative professionals, and athletic trainers who, by learning more about craniosacral therapy, will be better able to make appropriate referrals for craniosacral treatment. Craniosacral therapy training is also made available to a broad range of practitioners such as osteopathic physicians, medical doctors, doctors of oriental medicine, naturopathic physicians, dentists, psychiatrists, psychologists, physical therapists, occupational therapists, doctors of chiropractic, nurses, acupuncturists, massage therapists, and other such professionals. Contact Upledger Institute at 1-800-233-5880, Ext. 90012 or visit their Web site at <www.upledger.com>.

Each state has its own laws regarding licensure and for which patients or and in which health care settings treatment is appropriate. Therapists are required to practice under the laws of their own state, and health care professionals that use craniosacral therapy must be licensed or certified in a formal accredited health care profession.

Training Sites/Schools in Craniosacral Therapies

The Academy of Bio-Cranial Resonance
Info@cranialresonance.com

The College of Cranio-Sacral Therapy
9 St. George's Mews
Primrose Hills
London, England NW18XE
Phone: 020-7483-0120
E-mail: info@ccst.co.uk

The College of Osteopathic Medicine
Michigan State University
A314 East Fee Hall
East Lansing, Michigan 48824-1316
Phone: 517-353-0616
http://www.com.msu.edu/

Colorado School of Energy Studies
1721 Redwood Ave.
Boulder, Colorado 80304
Phone: 303-443-9847
http://www.energyschool.com
E-mail: info@energyschool.com

The Craniosacral Therapy Association of UK
Monomark House
27 Old Gloucester St.
London, England WC1N 3XX
Phone: 07000-784-735
E-mail: office@craniosacral.co.uk

Craniosacral Therapy Educational Trust
78 York Street
London, England W1H 1DP
Phone/Fax: 07000-785778
E-mail: infor@cranio.co.uk

The European School of Craniosacral Therapy
Alicante, Spain

The Institute of Craniosacral Studies
Phone: 0118-96-3986

Craniosacral Therapy Resources

The Upledger Institute
11211 Prosperity Farms Road
Palm Beach Gardens, Florida 33410-3487
1-800-233-5880, Ext. 90012
<www.upledger.com>

The Upledger Institute is a health resource center that is recognized worldwide for groundbreaking continuing education programs, clinical research, and therapeutic services using craniosacral therapy. The Institute was developed to educate the public and health care practitioners about the benefits of craniosacral therapy. It conducts hundreds of workshops around the world each year. It is a charitable organization that helps with research and development of innovative avenues of therapy that enable individuals to achieve their greatest levels of health and well-being. The Foundation provides community outreach, intensive therapy programs, and financial assistance to those in need.

For persons seeking craniosacral therapy, the Upledger Institute maintains the HealthPlex Clinic at the Florida facility. The Upledger Institute's HealthPlex Clinic is an innovative clinic that offers both private sessions and unique intensive therapy programs that address such conditions as migraine headaches, traumatic brain and spinal cord injuries, chronic neck and back pain, emotional difficulties, motor-coordination impairments, stress- and tension-related problems, central nervous system disorders, temporomandibular joint dysfunctions, orthopedic problems, chronic fatigue, scoliosis, neurovascular and immune disorders, infantile disorders, colic, post-traumatic stress disorder, autism, postsurgical dysfunctions, learning disabilities, fibromyalgia, and other connective tissue disorders. Contact number: 407-622-4706.

The Upledger Foundation's Brain and Spinal Cord Dysfunction Center offers a two-week intensive therapy program to individuals in need of rehabilitation and life-quality enhancement. At the center, patients and their caregivers receive sound advice and realistic hope. Contact number: 407-622-4706.

John Upledger, DO, FAAO, was the developer of craniosacral therapy. He is an osteopathic physician and surgeon. John E. Upledger is a recognized leader worldwide in the field of complementary health care, known for his many therapeutic innovations including establishment of the nonprofit Upledger Foundation, devoted to ongoing research and patient financial support, and services. He is on the Alternative Medicine Program Advisory Council for the Office of Alternative Medicine at the National Institutes of Health.

To find a qualified craniosacral therapist in your own area, Upledger's International Association of Healthcare Practitioners (IAHP) Web site at <www.iahp.com> lists professionals' telephone numbers, e-mail addresses, and levels of training. You can find a practitioner closest to your location and who would best be able to treat you. Copies of the directory are available by calling 1-800-233-5880 or 561-622-4334.

Beyond the Dura International Research Conference, sponsored by The Upledger Foundation, is offered semiannually. Contact number: 1-800-233-5880 or 407-624-3888.

Workshops are offered in the United States, Europe, and Asia: Contact 1-800-233-5880, ext. 44 or 561-622-4334.

Workshops concerning craniosacral therapy available from the Upledger Institute are as follows:

- Introduction to Craniosacral Therapy
- Craniosacral Therapy I
- Craniosacral Therapy II
- SomatoEmotional Release I
- SomatoEmotional Release II
- Advanced Craniosacral Therapy I
- Advanced Craniosacral Therapy II
- Applying Acupuncture Principles to Craniosacral Therapy

- Clinical Application of Craniosacral Therapy and SomatoEmotional Release
- Craniosacral Therapy for Pediatrics
- Craniosacral Therapy and the Immune Response
- Clinical Application of Advanced Craniosacral Therapy and Pediatrics
- The Brain Speaks
- Facial Mobilization I
- Muscle Energy I
- Muscle Energy II
- Visceral Manipulation I-A
- Visceral Manipulation I-B
- Visceral Manipulation II
- Practical Integration of Visceral Integration
- Advanced Visceral Manipulation
- Applying Acupuncture Principles to Bodywork

For a complete list of courses refer to <www.upledger.com/class/default .htm>.

Articles, Publications, and Books

Jean-Pierre Barral (1989). *Visceral Manipulation II*. Seattle: Eastland Press.
Jean-Pierre Barral and Pierre Mercier (1988). *Visceral Manipulation*. Seattle: Eastland Press.
John Basmajian (1975). *Grant's Method of Anatomy*. Baltimore, MD: Williams and Wilkins.
Gray's Anatomy, 35th British Edition. (1973). Philadelphia, PA: WB Saunders & Co.
Ernest Retzlaff, Fred Mitchell Jr., John Upledger, and Thomas Biggert (1978). Nerve Fiber and Endings in Cranial Sutures. *Journal of American Osteopathic Association*, 77 (February): 607.
Carolyn Reuben (1987). Craniosacral Therapy. *LA Weekly*, April 24-20.
John Upledger (1978). The Relationship of Craniosacral Examination Findings in Grade School Children with Developmental Problems. *Journal of American Osteopathic Association*, 77: 760169-774183.
John Upledger (1979). Mechano-Electric Patterns During Craniosacral Osteopathic Diagnosis and Treatment. *Journal of the American Osteopathic Association*, 78 (July): 78249-79158.
John Upledger (1980). Cranial Therapy Proves Successful with Some DD Children. *Association for Retarded Citizens Advocate*, January/February: 1.
John Upledger (1987). *Craniosacral Therapy II: Beyond the Dura*. Seattle: Eastland Press, Inc.

John Upledger (1989). The Facilitated Segment. *Massage Therapy Journal,* summer: 22-25.
John Upledger (1990). *SomatoEmotional Release and Beyond.* Palm Beach, FL: UI Publishing.
John Upledger (1997). *Your Inner Physician and You.* Berkley, CA: North Atlantic Books; Palm Beach Gardens, FL: UI Enterprises.
John Upledger and ZVI Karni (1979). Mechano-Electric Pattern During Craniosacral Osteopathic Diagnosis and Treatment. *Journal of American Osteopathic Association,* 78 (July): 782.
John Upledger and Jon Vredevoogd (1983). *Craniosacral Therapy.* Seattle: Eastland Press.

REFERENCES

Barnes, J. (1990). *Myofascial Release: The Search for Excellence: A Comprehensive Evaluatory and Treatment Approach.* Paoli, PA: Rehab Services, Inc.
Bodeau, J. (2002). Craniosacral Therapy: Unwinding the Soul. Available at <www.alaskawellness.com/bodyworkcraniosacral/archives.html>.
Breggin, P. (2002). Empathic Self Transformation in Therapy. In P. Breggin, G. Breggin, and F. Bernak (Eds.), *Dimensions of Empathic Therapy* (pp. 177-189). New York: Springer Publishing Company.
Burget, F.L. (2002). Craniosacral Therapy, A Hands-On Approach, May Help Restore Health. *Advance for Directors in Rehabilitation,* 67-70.
Burke, N. (1997). Beyond the Dura. Presentation at The Upledger Foundation Conference, San Diego, California, October.
Cohen, D.D.C. (1989a). The Craniosacral Rhythmic Impulse. *The American Chiropractor,* March 1.
Cohen, D.D.C. (1989b). The Nature of Palpation. *The American Chiropractor,* March 1.
Cohen, D.D.C. (1989c). Palpation of Craniosacral Motion. *The American Chiropractor,* March 1.
Cox, D. (2002). The Physical Body in Spiritual Formation: What God Has Joined Together Let No One Put Asunder. *Journal of Psychology and Christianity, 21* (3): 281-291.
Danese, S. (1989). Health and Fitness: Craniosacral Therapy. *Toronto New Age Monthly, 4* (2).
Gerome, S. (1997). Dialogue, Imagery, Craniosacral Therapy and Synchronicity. *Upledger Update.* Available at: <http://www.kineesis.com/html/cranio-genome.html>.
Glaser, A. (2002). The Alchemy of Compassion. Dissertation Abstracts International: Section B, *The Sciences & Engineering, 63* (5-6).
Heinrich, S. (1989). Learning to Let Go—The Role of Somato Emotional Release in Clinical Treatment. *Physical Therapy Forum, 13* (24).

Heinrich, S. (1991a). The Role of Physical Therapy in Craniofacial Pain Disorders: An Adjunct to Dental Pain Management. *The Journal of Craniomandibular Practice, 9* (1): 71-75.

Heinrich, S. (1991b). Toward an Understanding of Craniosacral Therapy. *Physical Therapy Forum, 10* (13).

Hutch, R. (2000). Character and Cure: "Patient, Heal Thyself." *Pastoral Psychology, 49* (2): 147-164.

Linley, A.P. and Joseph, S. (2003). Trauma and Personal Growth. *Psychologist, 16* (3): 135.

Nolen-Hoeksema, S. and Davis, C.G. (2002). Positive Responses to Loss, Perceiving Benefits and Growth. *Handbook of Positive Psychology,* 598-606.

Persaud, S.M. (2002). Dissertation Abstracts International: Section A, *Humanities & Social Sciences, 63* (1-A): 99.

Retzlaff, E., Mitchell, F., Upledger, J.E., and Biggert, T. (1978). Nerve Fibers and Endings in Cranial Structures. *Journal of American Osteopathic Association,* 77.

Retzlaff, E., Roppel, R., Becker, R.F., Mitchell, F., and Upledger, J.E. (1976). Craniosacral Mechanisms. *Journal of American Osteopathic Association,* 76.

Retzlaff, E., Upledger, J.E., Mitchell, F., and Walsh, J. (1979). Aging of Cranial Sutures in Humans. *The Anatomical Record, 193* (3).

Reuben, C. (1987). Health: Craniosacral Therapy. *L.A. Weekly.*

Rizzuto, A.M. (2003). Psychoanalysis: The Transformation of the Subject by the Spoken Word. *Psychoanalytic Quarterly, 72* (2): 287-323.

Sims, D. (1989). Headache: Successful Treatment of a Patient with Referred Symptom Headaches Utilizing Functional Motion Exercises and Soft Tissue Mobilization. *Orthopaedic Practice, 1* (4): 335-338.

Smoley, R. (1991). Bodywork: Exploring Craniosacral Therapy. *Yoga Journal,* 20(38): 20-29.

Upledger, J.E. (1978). The Relationship of Craniosacral Examination Findings in Grade School Children with Developmental Problems. *Journal of American Osteopathic Association,* 77: 760169-774183.

Upledger, J.E. (1980). Cranial Therapy Proves Successful with Some DD Children. *Association for Retarded Citizens Advocate Newsletter.* Lansing, MI: Greater Lansing Association for Retarded Citizens.

Upledger, J.E. (1983). Craniosacral Function on Brain Dysfunction. *Osteopathic Annals* (July): 9-12.

Upledger, J.E. (1996). In the Nick of Time. *Upledger Update,* p. 7.

Upledger, J.E. (1997). *Your Inner Physician and You.* Palm Beach Gardens, FL: North Atlantic Books and UI Enterprises.

Upledger, J.E. and Karni, Z. (1979a). Early Steps of Cranial Therapy in Israel. Available at <http://www.upledger.com/news/article/htm>.

Upledger, J.E. and Karni, Z. (1979b). Mechano-Electric Patterns During Craniosacral Osteopathic Diagnosis and Treatment. *Journal of American Osteopathic Association,* 78: 782149-791158.

Upledger, J.E. and Vredevoogd, J.D. (1983). *Craniosacral Therapy.* Chicago: Eastland Press.

West, W. (2001). Issues Relating to the Use of Forgiveness in Counselling and Psychotherapy. *British Journal of Guidance & Counselling, 29* (4): 415-428.

Wethington, E. (2003). Flourishing: Positive Psychology and the Life Well Lived. *American Psychological Association, 37*(53).

Workman, D. (2002). The Process of Psychospiritual Maturation in Adult-Acquired Severe Physical Disability: A Grounded Theory. Dissertation Abstracts International: Section B, *The Sciences & Engineering, 62* (10-B): 4505.

Index

Page numbers followed by the letter "f" indicate figures; those followed by the letter "t" indicate tables.